Supporting People Living With HIV

Mohd Rashid

Abstract

The HIV/AIDS epidemic, now in its fifth decade, is one of the most consequential health, social, scientific, and political challenges of the modern era. Since its emergence, social work has played a critical role in service provision and advocacy on behalf of people living with HIV/AIDS (PLWHA). Tremendous biomedical advancements over the years have fundamentally transformed HIV from an invariably fatal illness to a chronic and manageable condition. As the profile of HIV has changed over time, less is known about the contemporary experiences of social workers engaged with PLWHA. To address this gap, semi-structured interviews were conducted with early career social workers engaged with PLWHA (n = 22). Data were analyzed using interpretative phenomenological analysis (IPA). A modified socioecological model, complemented by life course theory, provides the conceptual framework informing the research process. Findings are organized along the five domains of the socioecological model—individual; interpersonal; organizational; community; and policy and societal. Three unifying themes emerge: making meaning of HIV; social work in the shadows of uncertainty; and HIV as a social work lens. The study explores how early career social workers construct professional identity, make sense of their work and the epidemic, and navigate personal, interpersonal, and structural challenges within shifting biomedical and policy landscapes. Implications, limitations, and strengths are addressed.

Table of Contents

Chapter 1
Introduction

Social workers who engage with people living with HIV/AIDS (PLWHA) play a vital role in the response to one of the greatest public health crises of the last century. While mostly confined to hospitals in the earliest years of the epidemic[1] (Willinger & Rice, 2003), social work with PLWHA today takes place in therapy offices, youth drop-in centers, substance use agencies, community mental health spaces, specialized outpatient clinics, and just about any location where clients[2] receive social and medical services. There are an estimated 1.2 million PLWHA in the United States, while over 30,000 individuals are infected with the virus every year (CDC, 2024). HIV continues to disproportionately affect marginalized communities, including sexual and racial minorities and low-income individuals (Lightfoot et al., 2021; Menza et al., 2021; Sullivan et al., 2021). PLWHA have lower health quality of life and greater prevalence of mental health conditions and substance use compared to the general population (Cook et al., 2018; Cooper et al., 2017; Yehia et al., 2015). Material deprivation, including housing insecurity and poverty, is common for PLWHA and contributes to poor health outcomes (Marcus et al., 2016; Oldenburg et al., 2014). Stigma and discrimination aimed at PLWHA have deleterious social, economic, and health consequences (Beer et al., 2022; Land & Linsk, 2013; Rice et al., 2018). In this fifth decade of the epidemic, sustained, well-funded, and comprehensive psychosocial interventions are still necessary to address the needs of PLWHA (Beyrer et al., 2021; Bowleg et al., 2022; Broz et al., 2021).

In many cases, social work practice with PLWHA may be indistinguishable from work with other client populations. However, HIV is uniquely situated within a complex environment characterized by social, political, medical, and moral conflicts social workers must navigate. At the onset of the epidemic, the virus was closely associated with sexual behaviors, substance use, and oppressed communities, contributing to a social response characterized by ignorance, stigma, and discrimination (Jones & Salazar, 2016; Merson et al., 2008). The stark images of people wasting away from AIDS-related complications crystalized the belief that HIV equated illness and death (Small, 1992; Varas-Díaz & Toro-Alfonso, 2003). The ferocity of the epidemic heightened difficult ethical issues, including debates about mandatory testing, duty to warn, and the limits of confidentiality (Dhai & Noble, 2005; Reamer, 1988, 1991). Fears of the virus and moral objections to PLWHA contributed to ineffective political responses, especially during the earliest years (Padamsee, 2017, 2020). As a counterweight to governmental inertia, grassroots activism and social service programs flourished that played an essential role in altering the trajectory of the epidemic (Emmer, 2012; Goldberg, 2022; Schulman, 2021). Determined and dramatic efforts on behalf of PLWHA and those most vulnerable to infection spurred unprecedented scientific achievements and led to medical treatments that transformed HIV/AIDS from an inevitably fatal disease to a chronic and manageable condition (Maeda et al., 2019; Palmisano & Vella, 2011). While a cure does not currently exist and the epidemic is not over, continued advancements in medication and science offer hope that the end of HIV may be closer than ever (Borrajo, 2025; Jin & Zhang, 2025; Lanzafame et al., 2025; Read et al., 2022).

Medications alone, in the absence of robust social services to support PLWHA, are insufficient to bring the epidemic to a conclusion. In 2019, the Ending the HIV

Epidemic (EHE) Initiative was launched to scale up the response to the virus. There are four pillars of this project: diagnose new cases of HIV as soon as possible after infection; treat PLWHA rapidly to achieve viral suppression; prevent new infections; and respond quickly to emerging clusters of new infections (Fauci et al., 2019). Social workers and other helping professionals, closely collaborating with medical providers, are charged to build new programs and strategies and maintain existing ones to achieve these goals. Beyrer and colleagues (2021) use a socioecological model to elucidate the multi-system and multi-level challenges to implementation of EHE that focuses on individual-level factors and considers how interpersonal networks, discrimination and stigma based upon HIV status, race, sexual orientation, and gender identity at the community level, and structural factors such as inadequate healthcare coverage and laws that further marginalize vulnerable populations serve as barriers to the eradication of HIV. Safe and affordable housing, accessible and affirming healthcare and mental health/substance use treatment, education and awareness programs about HIV, and policies that afford PLWHA and other marginalized individuals dignity and equity are some of the requirements to promote healthier and more stable lives, which should continue the downward trend of new infections to a point when society can truly celebrate the end of HIV.

However, the social services infrastructure that has sustained PLWHA is under attack and may be unable to meet current challenges. As the epidemic has changed, organizations that serve PLWHA have shifted priorities or discontinued operations. The AIDS Fund, one of Philadelphia's oldest and most respected AIDS service organizations (ASO) that raised over $18 million to support PLHWA, closed its doors in December 2024; leaders stated, "with the advances in both prevention and treatment we can conclude our work at this time" (Day, 2024). AIDS Walk Philly, a long-running fundraiser previously hosted by the AIDS Fund, has been retired by its successor sponsor, citing "rising costs, limited resources, and the shifting landscape of HIV awareness and funding" (Valdala, 2025). From Virginia to Washington State and many states in between, ASOs have ceased operations because of financial stress, even in areas that have seen an increase in new diagnoses (Holmes, 2024; Saunders, 2025). In the summer of 2024, two ASOs in Minneapolis suddenly closed within weeks of each other, leaving both clients and staff with little notice (Hazzard & Dernbach, 2025). Budget impasses and so-called efficiency initiatives have jeopardized care and services for the most vulnerable in Alabama (Hawkins, 2025), resulted in furloughs and cut hours for ASO employees in North Carolina (Fernandez, 2025), frozen testing for sexually transmitted infections (STIs) in Texas (Hollingsworth, 2025), and suspended Ohio's HIV services (Comeriato, 2025). While some grants and services have been restored, gaps in programming may cause harmful discontinuation of care for PLWHA and lower morale for social workers and other helping professionals who may remain out-of-work for long periods. More recently, several states have tightened eligibility requirements for drug assistance programs that offer low-income individuals access to life-saving medications, potentially affecting tens of thousands of PLWHA (Mandavilli, 2026). At the international level, the United Nations announced that UNAIDS, the agency responsible for leading the international response to HIV, may sunset at the end of 2026 due to deep cuts in foreign aid under the second administration of U.S. President Donald Trump (Rigby, 2025). Unfortunately, inadequate funding and political infighting are persistent features of the social services landscape. The tragedy here is that while the end of the epidemic is within reach, the necessary resources to finish the job may be unavailable.

The aim of this book is to gain a better understanding of the state of the epidemic and social work through an exploration of the experiences of early career social workers engaged with PLWHA. I define "early career social workers" as individuals who are currently enrolled in a Master of Social Work (MSW) program (or its social work equivalent) or received their MSW or equivalent social work degree within the last ten years. In selecting this population of interest, I wanted to learn how individuals who did not practice during the worst years of the epidemic understand HIV and make meaning of their work in the present moment. There is an abundance of research that addresses the vulnerabilities of PLWHA and the social determinants of HIV—the social, environmental, and economic systems that shape health and the conditions of life (Beltran et al., 2022; Hogan et al., 2021; Karram et al., 2024; Menza et al., 2021). But the interventions required to translate this research into practice are resource-intensive and logistically challenging to implement (Hotton et al., 2025). We know that PLWHA require housing, healthcare, and social connection, just to name a few; we know far less about how social workers on the ground handle the enormous responsibilities to make these happen. Research focusing on how social workers perform their jobs can provide new insights into the opportunities and challenges of the work, offer guidance for ASOs and other organizations that implement services for PLWHA, and suggest strategies to support and maintain a healthy and equitable workforce.

I utilize a modified socioecological model (SEM), grounded in the lived experiences of early career social workers engaged with PLWHA, to examine how intersecting factors across multiple levels affect social work practice. Drawing upon developmental psychology and health promotion, SEM is an effective tool for researchers seeking to learn more about PLWHA (Jain et al., 2023; Ojukwu et al., 2023; Sell et al.,

2016). Social workers engaged with PLWHA must learn to provide competent, caring, and ethical social work while tending to multidimensional factors including the social worker's personal values and background, interpersonal relationships with clients, organizational constraints, stigma and discrimination at the community level, and political and societal trends that impact social work practice. The proposed SEM for this research project is not a neat and orderly nest of systems, but a dynamic series of elements that may come into conflict. For the early career social worker, their practice identity—the essence of who they strive to be as a social worker—is closely connected to their success in traversing and making sense of this challenging environment.

I supplement the use of SEM with life course theory, which draws attention to the timing and sequencing of professional development and highlights how social workers' early experiences with clients, organizations, and policy environments impact their evolving understanding of HIV, their work with clients, and the trajectory of their social work careers. These encounters occur at a critical stage of professional development when early career social workers are exposed to competing messages about the scope and significance of the epidemic that vary depending on generational position, personal identities, and prior experiences. Together, SEM and life course theory provide a spatiotemporal perspective for comprehending how early career social workers making meaning of HIV and learn social work within shifting practice contexts.

The research question at the heart of this book is: "What are the experiences of early career social workers engaged with PLWHA?". To answer this question, I completed an interpretative phenomenological analysis (IPA) project consisting of 22 intensive, semi-structured interviews conducted from December 2024 to April 2025. In Chapter 2, I present a book review that offers a brief history of the HIV epidemic and the social work response from the earliest years to present day. Then, I explore the theoretical bases of SEM and life course theory and offer the modified SEM informing the book. In Chapter 3, I give an overview of the methodology of my research. In Chapters 4-8, I describe the findings from the interviews, with each chapter dedicated to a specific domain of the conceptual framework. In Chapters 9-10, I conclude with a discussion of the findings, implications for social work education, practice, research, and policy, and an acknowledgment of limitations and strengths of the project.

Chapter 2

Book Review and Conceptual Framework

The HIV epidemic is a profound public health challenge that led to medical innovations, advocacy movements, and holistic social interventions. Social work has played a central role in addressing the psychosocial, structural, and ethical dimensions of the care of PLWHA. This chapter situates HIV within its historical context, addresses the current state of the epidemic, and examines the essential social work response. The socioecological model (SEM) and life course theory are introduced as conceptual frameworks supporting this book, stressing how practice environments are shaped by social workers' individual histories, relationships with clients and colleagues, and broader organizational, community, historical, and social forces.

A Brief History of HIV/AIDS

In June 1981, a report in the Morbidity and Mortality Weekly Report (MMWR) noted an unusual cluster of five young men, "all active homosexuals", each of whom were stricken with a form of pneumonia only usually observed in individuals with severely compromised immune systems (Centers for Disease Control, 1981). The report states that two of the men reported "frequent homosexual contacts with various partners", while all five men disclosed inhalant drug use and one reported parenteral (i.e., IV-administered) drug use. In the editorial note, the authors surmise "[t]he fact that these patients were all homosexuals suggests an association between some aspect of a homosexual lifestyle or disease acquired through sexual contact and *Pneumocystis* pneumonia in this population." (Centers for Disease Control, 1981, p. 251). Within the year, hundreds more similar cases, mostly affecting gay men, were reported throughout the United States and other countries; researchers labeled this unexplained breakdown of the immune system as GRID (gay-related immunodeficiency) (Altman, 1982). In September 1982, the Centers for Disease Control[3] (CDC) first used the acronym AIDS (Acquired Immunodeficiency Syndrome) to describe this rapidly growing health crisis (Centers for Disease Control, 1982). Researchers identified other populations that experienced disproportionate numbers of AIDS diagnoses, including hemophiliacs, blood transfusion recipients, and intravenous (IV) drug users (Whiteside, 2016). Less than three years after the first identified cases, scientists discovered a causal link between a virus (later named the human immunodeficiency virus, or HIV) and AIDS (Gallo et al., 1984; Montagnier, 2002).

HIV is a retrovirus that converts its RNA into DNA and integrates this viral DNA into the genome of CD4 cells (white blood cells that coordinate the body's defense against pathogens), disrupting their function and ultimately contributing to their depletion (Redfield & Burke, 1988; Weber & Weiss, 1988; Whiteside, 2016). As HIV runs its course, it decimates more of the body's CD4 cells. The compromised immune system is easy prey to infections that would normally be obliterated by healthy CD4 cells (Bennett, 1986; Gallo & Montagnier, 1988). AIDS-related conditions may include pneumonia, fungal infections, Kaposi's sarcoma, lymphoma, meningitis, and tuberculosis. (Abrams, 1986; Holmberg & Meyer, 1986; Navarro & Kaplan, 2006; Wood & Harrington, 2005). A CD4 count below 200 cells/mm^3 is a CDC diagnostic criteria for AIDS (Li et al., 2023). Medical providers also look at the patient's viral load, or the amount of HIV material in a milliliter of blood (Drain et al., 2019; Saag et al., 1996). High viral loads (over 100,000 copies/mL) are often correlated with low CD4 counts (Gill et al., 2002; Phillips et al., 2001). By 1985, the Food and Drug Administration (FDA) licensed the first commercially available tests to screen for HIV, which proved to be an important turning point in the epidemic (Stoto et al., 1995).

It would take several years for scientists to make significant progress in the development of medications that would effectively manage HIV. The search for treatments was a tragic slog characterized by cycles of high expectations followed by dashed hopes (Sepkowitz, 2001). From 1981 to 1990, over 100,000 deaths were attributed to AIDS-related illness; by 1989, AIDS was estimated to be the second leading cause of death in men ages 25-44, surpassing heart disease, cancer, suicide, and homicide (Centers for Disease Control, 1991). Among those who died from AIDS during the first years of the epidemic, almost 60% occurred among gay and bisexual men and 21% among women and straight men who used IV drugs (CDC, 1991). From 1981-1982, 37% of the 400 AIDS cases were reported in individuals of minority races and ethnicities; that figure would explode to 72% by 2003 (Dean et al., 2005). Death rates continued to spike through the first half of the 1990s. In 1995, over 48,000 death certificates in the United States reported HIV infection as the cause of death (Selik et al., 2002). The estimated annual number of deaths among people with AIDS increased exponentially from 451 in 1981 to 50,628 in 1995 (Centers for Disease Control and Prevention, 2011). Deaths due to AIDS-related conditions were often painful, fearful, and isolated; medical and social service systems were ill-prepared for the devastation wrought by HIV (Brier, 2018; Daley, 1987). During this same period (1981-1995), the annual number of AIDS diagnoses grew rapidly, from 318 to 75,457 (CDC, 2011). Scientists estimate that between 628,000 to 988,000 Americans were infected with HIV as of January 1991 (Biggar & Rosenberg, 1993).

HIV is primarily transmitted through sexual contact, maternal-infant exposure (vertical transmission), and intravenous drug use (Forbes et al., 2012; Marks et al., 2022; Shaw & Hunter, 2012). The transmission occurs when bodily fluids that contain HIV make contact with mucous membranes and/or the bloodstream (Kull, 2010). In the earliest days of the epidemic, individuals also became infected through blood transfusions, which have the highest risk of transmission (Patel et al., 2014). Screening techniques have greatly reduced, but not eliminated, incidences of HIV transmission through blood transfusions (Scott & Wu, 2019). Condomless receptive anal intercourse is known to have a high risk of HIV transmission due to the rectal mucosa's susceptibility to the virus; researchers estimate the per-act of HIV transmission for insertive vaginal intercourse to be 4 per 10,000 exposures compared to 138 per 10,000 exposures for receptive anal intercourse (Kelley et al., 2017; Patel et al., 2014). Given the routes of transmission, certain populations have been disproportionately impacted by HIV. In the 1980s, these groups were derisively referred to as the "4-H Club": Homosexuals, Heroin users, Hemophiliacs, and Haitians (Fuchs & Leven, 2021; Marc et al., 2010). PLWHA were often grotesquely portrayed as unhealthy, deviant, and irresponsible purveyors of disease and death (Crawford, 1994; Mackereth, 1995; Mondragón et al., 1991).

PLWHA faced discrimination in housing, employment, and health care and were frequently shunned by friends and family (Gonsalves & Staley, 2014; Purcell, 2021). In one of the most infamous moments from the early years of the epidemic, three young brothers living with HIV required a federal court order to attend school in the face of vociferous protests and bomb threats; their home eventually burned to the ground with no perpetrator ever discovered (Esper, 1987). The commentator Willam Buckley (1986) called for a radical intervention in the pages of *The New York Times*: "Everyone detected with AIDS should be tattooed in the upper forearm, to protect common-needle users, and on the buttocks, to prevent the victimization of other homosexuals." Pat Buchanan (1983), who would go on to become White House Communications Director during the height of the epidemic, opined in *The New York Post*: "The poor homosexuals. They have declared war on nature, and now nature is exacting an awful retribution." Attitudes and beliefs about HIV and PLWHA were deeply rooted in misinformation and homophobia. In one study, 53% of male respondents and 51% of female respondents agreed with the statement: "I don't feel sorry for drug abusers who catch AIDS because it is their own fault", while 52% of males and 44% of females concurred that: "I don't feel sorry for homosexuals who catch AIDS because it is their own fault" (Nutbeam et al., 1989). In another study, 74% of participants would not eat in a restaurant with a kitchen worker with AIDS and 71% of participants would not kiss someone with AIDS on the cheek (Stipp & Kerr, 1989). The authors of this second study found that attitudes about gay people, not education level, were the strongest individual predictor of beliefs about HIV (Stipp & Kerr, 1989).

The initial response to the epidemic by federal, state, and local governments, with some notable exceptions, was plodding, haphazard, and inadequate to meet the moment. In October 1982, a reporter asked White House Press Secretary Larry Speakes the first ever question about the growing epidemic during a press briefing. Speakes claimed ignorance about AIDS and jokingly asked the reporter if he had HIV (Ortiz, 2023). President Ronald Reagan first acknowledged HIV publicly in 1985, shortly after his friend, actor Rock Hudson, announced that he was living with HIV (Richert, 2009). It would not be until 1987, at the urging of his wife Nancy, that Reagan gave his first speech about HIV (Tumulty, 2021). Consistent with his belief in limited government, Reagan cut budgets at agencies such as National Institutes of Health (NIH) and CDC and surrounded himself with social conservatives who possessed dim views of the individuals most susceptible to HIV infection (Padamsee, 2020). The dithering amidst the despair was a bipartisan affair. Mayor Ed Koch, a Democrat from New York City, one of the epicenters of the HIV epidemic, was pilloried for his failures to meet with community members and direct sufficient resources to PLWHA; by January 1984, with almost 900 dead of AIDS, the city spent a total of $24,500 in response (France, 2013). By contrast, Mayor Dianne Feinstein of San Francisco chaired the first national task force devoted to AIDS through the U.S. Conference of Mayors and was widely praised (despite some notable missteps) for her pioneering efforts to build public and private networks of HIV-related care and services that would become known as the "San Francisco Model" (Feinstein, 1987; Roberts, 2023). However, principled and effective leadership was in short supply within government. Responsibility fell upon citizen-activists to fight for the rights and needs of PLWHA.

The sclerotic governmental response highlighted that HIV was not just a health crisis, but a political crisis as well (Brier, 2018). While some leaders called for quarantines and other isolative strategies, it was apparent such measures would be futile because of the distinctive nature of the virus and the social vulnerabilities of individuals most impacted by the epidemic (Smith & Whiteside, 2010). Such harsh interventions would have driven the epidemic further underground, making it more challenging to address (Rosenbrock et al., 2000). Grassroots organizations, often founded and led by PLWHA, sprouted up to address the overwhelming medical and social emergency. In

1982, Gay's Men's Health Crisis in New York City, AIDS Project Los Angeles, and San Francisco AIDS Foundation were founded, while existing organizations such as Whitman-Walker Clinic in Washington, D.C. and Howard Brown Health Center in Chicago repurposed their missions to address the epidemic; this was the beginning of an AIDS service industry that is still in force today (Brier, 2018; Parker, 2010). While these organizations offered crucial aid during the darkest days, their objectives were often myopically focused on the needs of gay White men. Queer people of color built organizations, such as BEBASHI in Philadelphia and Third World AIDS Advisory Taskforce in San Francisco, to address racially disparate outcomes and treatment (Brier, 2018; Royles, 2020). These AIDS service organizations (ASOs) offered medical support for PLWHA and provided a host of services, including housing, social connections and activities, meals for homebound individuals, and case management (Chambre, 1997; Thompson, 2014). While public agencies would eventually assume a more prominent role in addressing HIV, these grassroots ASOs provided an exceptional level of care (Chambre, 1997).

During the initial years of the epidemic, there were considerable disagreements among activists whether their energy should be devoted to service provision or deployed to larger-scale advocacy (Parker, 2010; Schulman, 2021). In 1987, the group ACT UP (AIDS Coalition to Unleash Power) was founded in New York as a "diverse, non-partisan group of individuals, united in anger and committed to direct action to end the AIDS crisis" (Schulman, 2021, p. v). Schulman (2021) states that direct action was essential to ACT UP's mission: "[t]he differentiation between direct action and social services was rooted in an understanding that activists created change that required policy, and social service providers, and later AIDS Incorporated professionals, institutionalized and carried out policy." (p. 28). However, the divide between direct action and social service provision was not as binary. ACT UP's campaign for needle exchange programs revolutionized harm reduction and the ACT UP Housing Committee would eventually transform into Housing Works, one of the nation's premier ASOs (Schulman, 2021).

ACT UP and its sibling affiliates throughout the country engaged in a wide range of direct action designed to motivate, cajole, and shame individuals in positions of power and authority to sufficiently address the HIV epidemic. ACT UP's overarching strategy consisted of two distinct yet complementary dynamics. ACT UP members became infamous for their displays of civil disobedience, designed to attract maximum attention and generate maximum outrage, including well-publicized protests inside St. Patrick's Cathedral, Shea Stadium (former home of the New York Mets), and the storming of NIH headquarters in Bethesda, MD, to name just a few (Brier, 2018; Gamson, 1989; Schulman, 2021). The presence of ACT UP in New York City was enhanced by cultural and artistic activism, including posters, stickers, and T-shirts whose messages (such as SILENCE=DEATH) became the movement's calling cards (Burk, 2015). By contrast, other members of ACT UP developed relationships with regulators at the FDA and other political appointees to drive change and spur scientific innovation from inside the halls of power (Richert, 2009; Schulman, 2021). For many members of ACT UP, their overarching concern was getting "drugs into bodies", which at times left little appetite to address other issues such as racism, sexism, and classism both within and outside of the movement (Stockdill, 2013). While the urgency was understandable, the tensions between different factions within ACT UP, combined with fatigue and a steady increase in deaths, led to schisms that ultimately diminished the movement (Denton et al., 2022; Schulman, 2021; Stockdill, 2013).

The course of the HIV epidemic took a dramatic turn in the 1990s with the development of antiretroviral therapies (ART). ART consists of a medication regimen, often a combination of different types of drugs, that interferes with HIV replication at critical stages, thereby limiting the progression of the virus (Aquaro et al., 2020; Shin et al., 2021; Voshavar, 2019). The suppression of HIV results in lower viral loads, increased CD4 cells, and enhanced immune systems (Phillips et al., 2001; Shoko & Chikobvu, 2019). ART is not a cure for HIV; PLWHA must carefully adhere to medication regimens for their intended effect (Beer & Skarbinski, 2014; Robbins et al., 2014). ART gave life and hope to PLWHA, transforming the virus from an acute and invariably fatal malady to a chronic and manageable condition (Marins et al., 2003; Oguntibeju, 2012). Deaths and opportunistic infections declined rapidly, while the life expectancy of PLWHA dramatically increased (Marcus et al., 2016; Palella et al., 1998). The dramatic change in the trajectory of the epidemic inspired hope that the end was in sight (Sullivan, 1996), but HIV was not eradicated. An estimated 40,907 new cases were reported in 1999, increasing to 41,113 the following year (Klevens & Neal, 2002). With PLWHA living longer, the prevalence of AIDS steadily increased over time; by end of 2000, there were an estimated 337,731 PLWHA in the United States (Klevens & Neal, 2002). By 2008, there was an estimated 1.18 million PLWHA, 20% of whom were not yet diagnosed (Chen et al., 2012).

ART only works for PLWHA if they have access to the medications, which proved prohibitively expensive for most individuals. Medicaid, which covers the cost of ART, is the single largest source of insurance for PLWHA; approximately 40% of PLWHA are covered by this program (Dawson et al., 2025). 28% of PLWHA are covered by Medicare; the addition of the Part D benefit in 2006 designated ART as a protected drug class, although some enrollees may share in the cost of their medications (Dawson et al., 2023). AIDS Drug Assistance Programs (APAP), which began in 1987 and are now incorporated into the Ryan White CARE Program, provide free medications for individuals not covered by government or private insurance (Hanna et al., 2013; Ludema et al., 2016). But, evoking one of ACT UP's mantras, the challenge remained how to get drugs into bodies. While many PLWHA successfully adapted to daily medication routines, consistent ART use was difficult for many. Studies at the time suggest that between 40-60% of individuals were less than 90% adherent[4], and that adherence generally decreases over time (Bartlett, 2002). Individuals struggling with substance use, mental health conditions, lower cognitive functioning due to aging, and unstable housing have more trouble with adherence (Hinkin et al., 2002; Rabkin & Chesney, 1999; Roberts & Mann, 2000; Sorensen et al., 1998). Initial ART schedules could be burdensome. PLWHA might have to take anywhere up to two dozen or more pills at different times throughout the day. Some medications had to be refrigerated and taken with food, which could be challenging for people of limited means (Bamberger et al., 2000; Chesney et al., 2000; Franco et al., 2002). While medication nonadherence is a problem that predates the epidemic (Chesney, 2006; Wright, 2000), this issue received greater attention from researchers and providers.

With the introduction of ART, there was an important shift in public opinion and policymaking (Scandlyn, 2000). As deaths declined in the United States, press coverage of the epidemic on the domestic front waned while there was a substantial increase in attention overseas, suggesting HIV was someone else's problem (Stevens & Hull, 2013). As the prevalence of HIV increased due to longer life expectancy, federal dollars did not keep up with the considerable costs of medical care and social supports (Martin &

Keenan, 2011). PLWHA who were once resigned to die now had to learn how to cope with unexpected survival (Brashers et al., 1999; Owen & Catalan, 2012). Living with a chronic medical condition comes with physical, emotional, and financial challenges, while the management of the condition "increasingly falls on the shoulders of those who have the illness. In the absence of a crisis, it is easy to forget that people with an illness are still working hard to care for themselves and to resume what could now constitute a normal life." (Scandlyn, 2000, p. 133).

ART has substantially improved since its introduction in the mid-1990s. Today, ART is considered safe, highly efficacious, and relatively easy to administer; several therapies now consist of one multi-drug pill taken daily (Airoldi et al., 2010; Choudhary & Mellors, 2022; Masters et al., 2019). However, consistent adherence remains a problem for many PLWHA (Freeman et al., 2021; Whiteley et al., 2021). Long-acting injectable ART holds great promise for individuals who struggle with daily maintenance; such regimens may require an injection monthly, every other month, or twice a year (Brizzi et al., 2023; Wang et al., 2023). Medical providers face barriers to the uptake of injectables at drug-level (drug resistance, drug-drug interactions), patient-level (perceived side effects, frequency of injections, medical mistrust, fear of needles), and system-level (training and education for providers, additional strain on overburdened clinics) (Cooper et al., 2022; Palacios et al., 2022).

ART adherence has taken on even greater urgency in the most recent years of the epidemic. Multiple studies show that PLWHA who are medication adherent and virally suppressed (<200 copies/mL) are highly unlikely to transmit the virus to someone not living with HIV (Bavinton et al., 2018; Cohen et al., 2011; Rodger et al., 2019). This has led to the U=U movement, a campaign that emphasizes that PLWHA who are undetectable (i.e., virally suppressed) cannot transmit the virus to their sexual partners (Bekker et al., 2023; Eisinger et al., 2019). This crucial discovery is the linchpin of Treatment as Prevention (TasP), a strategy for maximizing medication adherence and viral suppression as the primary method of stopping new infections (Delva et al., 2012; Hull & Montaner, 2013). Important elements of TasP include identifying PLWHA who are unaware of their status and connecting them with care, re-engaging PLWHA who have fallen out of the HIV continuum of care, and achieving viral suppression among those in care (Bernays et al., 2021; Delva et al., 2012). Another significant development was the discovery that consistent ART use can protect individuals not living with HIV from become infected with the virus; this strategy is known as pre-exposure prophylaxis (PrEP) (Donnell et al., 2014; Spinner et al., 2016). These biomedical advancements offer hope that the end of the epidemic is closer than ever (Fauci et al., 2019; Giroir, 2020). In 2010, the Obama Administration released the first comprehensive National HIV/AIDS Strategy (updated in 2015) that re-dedicated the nation to minimizing new infections, improving access to care, and reducing health disparities (Padamsee, 2020; Volansky et al., 2010; Yehia & Frank, 2011). The first Trump Administration issued its own plan in 2019 known as Ending the HIV Epidemic (EHE) that set out ambitious goals for eradicating the virus, including reducing new infections by 75% within five years and by 90% within ten years; Congress also approved $400 million dollars in new funding to support these efforts (Beyrer et al., 2021; Demeke et al., 2020; Schmid, 2021). There are concerns these targets will not be achieved in the desired time frames (Guilamo-Ramos et al., 2023). The first months of the second Trump Administration brought a series of challenges, including withdrawals from international health organizations, terminations of federal grants to support research relevant to HIV and PLWHA, anticipated budgetary and Medicaid cuts, and the appointment of an HIV denialist as Secretary of Health and Human Services (Robert F. Kennedy, Jr.), to name but a few (Greer et al., 2025; Kalichman, 2025; Smith, 2025). Anyone interested in learning more about the current state of HIV in mid-2025 was greeted by the following statement on the CDC (2025) website:

> Per a court order, HHS is required to restore this website as of 11:59PM ET, February 14, 2025. Any information on this page promoting gender ideology is extremely inaccurate and disconnected from the immutable biological reality that there are two sexes, male and female. The Trump Administration rejects gender ideology and condemns the harms it causes to children, by promoting their chemical and surgical mutilation, and to women, by depriving them of their dignity, safety, well-being, and opportunities. This page does not reflect biological reality and therefore the Administration and this Department rejects it.

The following table (Table 1) offers a summary of major milestones in the HIV epidemic in the United States.

Table 1

Major Milestones in the HIV/AIDS Epidemic in the United States

Year	Event	Brief Description
1981	First CDC MMWR Report	CDC reports rare pneumonia cases among gay men in Los Angeles, marking the first official recognition of the epidemic (Centers for Disease Control, 1981).
1982	AIDS Term Adopted	CDC formally names the health condition that often accompanied HIV as Acquired Immune Deficiency Syndrome (Centers for Disease Control, 1982).
1983	HIV Identified	Researchers identified the virus responsible for AIDS, later named HIV (Gallo et al., 1984; Montagnier, 2002).

1985	First Antibody Test	Blood screening begins in the U.S., dramatically reducing transfusion-related transmission. (Stoto et al., 1995).
1987	AZT Approved	The U.S. Food and Drug Administration approves AZT, the first antiretroviral medication (D'Andrea et al., 2008).
1987	ACT UP Founded	Activists organized to demand faster drug approval, research equity, and federal accountability (Schulman, 2021).
1990	Ryan White CARE Act	Congress passes legislation named after Ryan White, expanding care for low-income PLWHA (Siplon, 1999).
1991	Red Ribbon Introduced	The red ribbon became an international symbol of HIV/AIDS awareness and solidarity (McDonnell et al., 2017).
1994	Perinatal Transmission Reduced	AZT shown to significantly reduce mother-to-child HIV transmission (Cohen, 1995).
1996	ART Introduced	Combination antiretroviral (ART) dramatically reduces HIV-related mortality (Aquaro et al., 2020).
2003	PEPFAR Established	The President's Emergency Plan for AIDS Relief launches, expanding U.S. global HIV leadership (Varmus, 2013).
2010	National HIV/AIDS Strategy	First comprehensive federal strategy to reduce HIV incidence and address disparities (Yehia & Frank, 2011).
2012	PrEP Approved	FDA approves Truvada for pre-exposure prophylaxis, marking a major prevention breakthrough (Donnell et al., 2014).
2013	U=U Scientific Consensus	Evidence confirms that undetectable viral load prevents sexual transmission (Calabrese & Mayer, 2019).
2015	Indiana HIV Outbreak	Rural outbreak linked to injection drug use highlights need for harm reduction infrastructure (Janowicz, 2016).
2019	Ending the HIV Epidemic Initiative	Federal initiative aims to reduce new infections by 90% by 2030 (Beyrer et al., 2021).
2020	COVID-19 Disruption	Pandemic significantly disrupts HIV testing, prevention, and treatment services (Jewell et al., 2020).
2021	Long-Acting Injectable ART	First long-acting ART therapy approved in the U.S. (Venkatesan, 2022).
2023	Long-Acting Injectable PrEP Expanded	Injectable prevention options broaden adherence possibilities (Liegeon & Ghosn, 2023).

The State of HIV Today

Even if new infections ended today, HIV would remain a serious health concern. There were almost 32,000 new diagnoses of HIV in the U.S. in 2022 (Kaiser Family Foundation, 2024a). An estimated 1.2 million individuals (.4% of population) in the U.S. are living with HIV, approximately 13% of whom are unaware of their status (Kaiser Family Foundation, 2024a). An estimated 57% of PLWHA in the U.S. are virally suppressed (Kaiser Family Foundation, 2024a). HIV continues to disproportionately impact already marginalized populations. By the end of 2022, an estimated 739,200 MSM[5] and 63,000 MSM and IDU[6] were living with HIV, accounting for 65% of all PLWHA (Centers for Disease Control and Prevention, 2024a). 70% of all new diagnoses in 2022 were among gay and bisexual men (Centers for Disease Control and Prevention, 2024b). Racial disparities continue to define the HIV epidemic. 40% of all PLWHA are Black (KFF, 2024b). While Black individuals represent approximately 12% of the U.S. population, they account for 39% of new HIV diagnoses (Kaiser Family Foundation, 2024b). In 2022, 50% of all diagnoses in young people (ages 13-24) were among Black people and 53% of all gay and bisexual young people with HIV were Black (Kaiser Family Foundation, 2024b) Rates of new diagnoses for Black individuals are about 8 times that of White people and twice that of Hispanics (Kaiser Family Foundation, 2024b). Hispanic individuals constitute 19% of the population but 31% of all new diagnoses and 26% of PLWHA (Kaiser Family Foundation, 2024c). While there was a 12% decrease in HIV diagnoses in the overall population from 2010-2022, there was a 24% increase in new diagnoses among Hispanic individuals (Kaiser Family Foundation, 2024c). 81% of new diagnoses among Hispanics involve male-to-male sexual contact (Kaiser Family Foundation, 2024c). Asian Americans have the lowest rates of HIV incidence and prevalence; in 2018, Asian Americans made up 6% of the U.S. population but only 2% of new diagnoses (Centers for Disease Control and Prevention, 2024d).

Since the beginning of the HIV epidemic, women have been affected by the virus, but their needs have not received the same attention as other impacted demographics and they have been underrepresented in research projects (Adimora et al., 2021; Barr et al., 2024; Watkins-Hayes, 2019). Women constitute 22% of PLWHA in the U.S. and account for 19% of all new diagnoses in 2022 (Kaiser Family Foundation, 2024d). Black women have the highest rate of new diagnoses (50%) among women (Kaiser Family Foundation, 2024d). Transgender individuals, who comprise approximately .3% of the U.S. population, accounted for 2% (671) of new diagnoses in 2019; nearly 81% were among Black and Hispanic individuals (Centers for Disease Control and Prevention, 2024c). Individuals who live in the U.S. South have higher rates of HIV incidence and prevalence and lower access to care compared to other geographic areas; these disparities may be due to lack of Medicaid expansion, fewer providers, lower health literary, and greater HIV stigma (Kimmel et al., 2018; Masiano et al., 2019; Sullivan et al., 2021). As PLWHA are living longer, the population is skewing older. Over 50% of PLWHA are over the age of 50, and by 2030 it is estimated that 70% of PLWHA will be over 50 (Marium et al., 2023; Wing, 2016).

PLWHA, even those who have achieved viral suppression, often experience greater health challenges, multimorbidity, and lower quality of life compared to individuals who are not living with HIV (Althoff et al., 2024; Lazarus et al., 2021; Miners et al., 2014). Tobacco, alcohol, and other substance use are more prevalent among PLWHA compared to the population at large; substance use has been found to contribute to HIV infection and complicate engagement with medical care and other support services

(Duko et al., 2019; Hoang et al., 2024; Khalsa et al., 2008; Pitpitan et al., 2023). PLWHA are at increased risk of a host of medical issues, including obesity, hypertension, stroke, cardiovascular disease, hepatitis C, and tuberculosis (Bailin et al., 2020; Bogorodskaya et al., 2019; Fahme et al., 2018; Hsue & Waters, 2019; Kwan & Ernst, 2011; Soriano et al., 2023). HIV infection is correlated with insulin resistance, while use of ART has been associated with type 2 diabetes (Noubissi et al., 2018). PLWHA have poorer health quality of life than the general population, even when controlling for viral suppression and overall immune system health. (Miners et al., 2014; Skogen et al., 2023). These health conditions can impede engagement with HIV care, worsening the overall outlook for PLWHA (Fuster- Ruiz de Apodaca et al., 2023; Lazarus et al., 2023).

PLWHA experience mental health challenges, including depression, anxiety, and suicidal ideations, at greater rates than in the general population (Catalan et al., 2011; Hoare et al., 2021; Remien et al., 2019; Xu et al., 2023). Trauma is a pervasive problem for many PLWHA. The Substance Abuse and Mental Health Services Administration (SAMHSA) states that trauma "results from an event, series of events, or set of circumstances that is experienced by an individual as physically or emotionally harmful or life threatening and that has lasting adverse effects on the individual's functioning and mental, physical, social, emotional, or spiritual well-being." (U.S. H.H.S., 2014, p. 7). Compared to the general population, PLWHA are disproportionately impacted by trauma and its aftermath (Brezing et al., 2015; LeGrand et al., 2015; Sales et al., 2016). Poor health outcomes, including increased viral loads and decreased CD4 counts, are associated with the presence of trauma in the lives of PLWHA (Glynn et al., 2019, 2021; Leserman, 2008). The etiologies of the trauma experienced by PLWHA occur at micro-, mezzo-, and macro-levels during all stages of human development. Childhood trauma and adverse childhood experiences (ACEs) are prevalent among PLWHA (Cuca et al., 2019; Wallace et al., 2020; Young-Wolff et al., 2019). Such trauma can result in an increased risk of substance use and condomless intercourse, which are highly correlated with HIV infection (Sassoon et al., 2023). Given the propensity for trauma, it is unsurprising that PLWHA experience higher rates of posttraumatic stress disorder (PTSD) when compared to the general population (Ayano et al., 2020; López et al., 2023; Neigh et al., 2016). The diagnosis of HIV can be a traumatic event in of itself (Mgbako et al., 2020). Stigma, discrimination, and interpersonal violence have negative effects on the wellbeing and quality of life of PLWHA (Fatoki, 2016; Kouyoumdjian et al., 2013; Pitasi et al., 2018a). PLWHA encounter structural racism and homophobia (Arnold et al., 2014a; Burton et al., 2023), as well as ineffective laws that unjustly criminalize HIV transmission (Hoppe, 2017; Purcell, 2021). While there have been considerable advancements in the treatment of HIV, there has not been the same level of innovation and attention to the trauma of PLWHA (Brown & Adeagbo, 2022).

Many PLWHA struggle with problems of daily living and subsistence. Compared to individuals who are not living with HIV, PLWHA face a greater array of psychosocial stressors, including poverty, housing insecurity, unemployment, food insecurity, and a lack of affordable and reliable transportation (Aidala et al., 2016; Conyers et al., 2017; Harrison et al., 2025; Kalichman et al., 2019; Weiser et al., 2009). These troubles can cause PLWHA to drop out of care, worsening health outcomes (Ham et al., 2023; Mendonca et al., 2022). The provision of support services that address the physical health, mental health, environmental challenges, and material needs of PLWHA is crucial to ensure their wellbeing (Miltz et al., 2025).

Social Work Response to HIV Epidemic

Parker (2000) describes HIV as the "quintessential epidemic of the late twentieth century" and states that the virus "has tended to uncover the fault lines of social cleavage—as well as the capacity (or incapacity) of different social, cultural, and political systems to respond to impeding disaster in more or less humane and efficacious ways." (p. 39). Similarly, HIV could be considered a quintessential social work issue at the turn of the millennium (Kaplan et al., 2004). The virus' vicious course, the disenfranchisement and stigmatization of PLWHA, the initial lack of resources and supports to address the epidemic, and the exploding death toll cried out for a prolonged, coordinated, and multidimensional response long associated with social work. Social work has a long and effective history of addressing matters pertaining to public health (Gehlert & Browne, 2011; Ruth & Marshall, 2017; Sable et al., 2012). From the earliest days of the epidemic, social workers have played an essential role in caring for PLWHA, their loved ones and communities, and the larger society. While the epidemic has changed, social work continues to make important contributions in the battle to eliminate HIV.

The Initial Response

Social work, with its historic emphasis on both the individual and their surrounding environment and ability to develop and deliver interventions, was particularly well-suited to address the HIV epidemic. Ryan (1988) argues that the social workers engaged with PLWHA have "two clients: the person and their environment. The ultimate fate of people with AIDS is inextricably linked with how they are perceived, responded to and cared for" (p. 4). The earliest forms of social work with PLWHA comprised two components: practical services and resources such as housing, connections to public assistance, and transportation; and emotional support in response to the diagnosis, illness, and death (Strom, 2012). Social workers developed intervention models to address the biopsychosocial consequences of the epidemic. Lopez and Getzel (1984) note that the nature of AIDS, unpredictable in its trajectory yet progressing toward a grim final outcome, made traditional problem-solving approaches extremely difficult. They state that the social worker is "caught in a powerful dilemma: on the one hand, supporting the patient in overcoming the immediate crisis that can be handled through problem-solving and provision of supportive services and, on the other, preparing the patient for a death which may occur at any time" (p. 390). Through their pioneering work with GMHC, Lopez and Getzel fashioned a social work approach that placed a primary emphasis on the emotional and material needs of the client, buttressed by social and family supports when possible. This crisis intervention model consisted of seven phases: engagement and assessment; supporting autonomy; explaining the relationship and meaning of AIDS; supporting the patient in indirect recognition of death; monitoring and maintaining health status; supporting close relationships and griefwork; and caring and advocating for the dying patient (Lopez & Getzel, 1984). These social workers emphasize that the epidemic was indeed a crisis, reflected in the name of their organization (Gay Men's Health Crisis). The crisis of HIV was the cumulative impact of multiple infections and illnesses that defied treatment and weakened the ability of clients to address various challenges. The crisis element of the work was often complicated by the nature of the client's relationships with family and friends, especially if they lived far away and/or were unfamiliar with the client's sexual orientation (Lopez & Getzel, 1984). Lopez and Getzel were hopeful that the epidemic "may serve as the basis for establishing more extensive services in regions with concentrated gay populations as well as more meaningful linkages to 'straight' health and social service organizations" (p. 394). Lopez died of AIDS-related complications in 1986 (The New York Times, 1986).

Christ and her colleagues (1986), social workers at Memorial Sloan-Kettering Cancer Center in New York City, developed a psychosocial intervention social work model for the care of PLWHA. They make explicit connections between the client's wellbeing and the conditions of their social environment, stating "[i]t was clear that activities designed to reduce emotional, social, and physical stress among AIDS patients and their caregivers and to foster public attitudes that facilitated patient management would result in more effective delivery of treatment and strengthen preventive efforts" (p. 176). Their model started with an orientation to their hospital setting and a psychosocial assessment, followed by ongoing interventions and supports for both the client and their support network (if any), group work, client education supplemented with printed materials, and frequent communication and collaboration with medical providers. These social workers believed that one of the positive consequences of the epidemic was the development of a social work practice that stressed the coordination and cooperation of medical systems, social service providers, government actors, and advocates for the gay community and drug users (Christ et al., 1986).

The multidimensional aspects of HIV/AIDS, and the need for interventions at all levels of human interaction, were recognized at the onset of the epidemic. Furstenberg and Meltzer Olson (1984) assert the epidemic "vividly demonstrate[s] a proposition that underlies all of social work in the health field, that health and health care are not just matters of biology and physiology, or of medicine and medical technology. The situation surrounding AIDS serves to bring into sharp relief the fact that every health condition, good health, illness and disability, is at once a physical, psychological, social, economic and political phenomenon" (pp. 47-48). They highlight the role of culture and identity as an essential element of working with PLWHA and observe that the client's sexual orientation can affect their response to their illness, including access to resources and willingness to engage with providers (Furstenberg & Meltzer Olson, 1984). They also stress that the social worker intervenes with multiple individuals and organizations beyond the client, including families and significant others, health care providers, community members, and policymakers. The social worker must draw upon different skills and strategies, all with "the goals of minimizing the negative impact of AIDS and of mobilizing the resources of individuals and institutions to deal with AIDS" (Furstenberg & Meltzer Olson, 1984, p.60). Furtstenberg and Meltzer Olson note that while social work with PLWHA necessarily addresses negative fears, prejudices, and attitudes about the virus and those living with it, social workers themselves are not immune to these feelings. Social workers "must examine and bring into consciousness their own attitudes, beliefs, and feelings, and the ways these affect their responses…[u]nderstanding their own negative reactions also allows social workers to be more attuned to the fears and defenses of others" (Furstenberg & Meltzer Olson, 1984, p. 60). Thus, self-awareness is a critical component of social work practice with PLWHA.

The social work response to the onset of the HIV epidemic was not universally affirming of PLWHA. Mantell and her colleagues (1989) reviewed the patient records for 152 PLWHA who were patients at one of New York City's largest hospitals during the first few years of the epidemic; they found that social workers provided services to only 40% of PLWHA. While they hypothesize that anxiety contributed to low levels of engagement, the authors did not specifically examine the psychosocial needs and concerns of hospital staff (Mantell et al., 1989). They note the heavy demands placed upon staff, lack of sufficient resources, and emotional toll produced by the work. The authors call for increased education and training for all providers working with PLWHA, in addition to dedicated resources and programs specifically tailored to address the concerns of PLWHA (Mantell et al., 1989).

Research during the first decade of the epidemic suggests that social workers and other helping professionals struggled with fears and prejudices about HIV and PLWHA. Numerous studies across different populations found a significant negative correlation between fear of AIDS, homophobic beliefs, and knowledge about HIV (Goodwin & Roscoe, 1988; Kelly et al., 1987; O'Mahony, 1989; Temoshok et al., 1987). Social workers and other helping professionals demonstrated similar attitudes. O'Donnell and colleagues (1987) surveyed 237 hospital social workers at a major hospital in Massachusetts. Respondents expressed fears and misconceptions about PLWHA. Almost three-quarters of their sample agreed that PLWHA should not be allowed to handle food in restaurants, while 42% agreed that a hospital worker should not be required to work with AIDS patients (O'Donnell et al., 1987). Homophobia was prevalent in this study; 43% of respondents would seek psychiatric treatment for their child if they learned they were gay, while almost half agreed that the thought of homosexual acts was disgusting. The authors find a positive correlation between AIDS phobia (including fear of contagion) and homophobia and stress about AIDS. They suggest training programs for hospital social workers not just concentrate on the medical facts about AIDS, but also offer emotional support to cope with the unknown elements of the virus and provide sensitization to issues of sexual orientation (O'Donnell et al., 1987).

Samuel and Boyle (1989) researched the attitudes, beliefs, and knowledge about AIDS among 87 social service providers (social workers, administrative aides, and paraprofessionals) to facilitate their planning of a training course on the epidemic. They found that homophobia and fear about AIDS were negatively correlated with knowledge about the virus (Samuel & Boyle, 1989). However, they were some significant differences between social workers and other providers. Social workers had more information, more positive attitudes, and more willingness to engage in certain behaviors (such as cleaning up the blood of PLWHA) than other providers (Samuel & Boyle, 1989). Age was also a significant factor; younger individuals had higher scores on all three measures of the scale (information, attitude, and behavior) and were more likely to have contact with family and friends who were gay (Samuel & Boyle, 1989).

Wiener and Siegel (1990) examined social workers' comfort in providing services to PLWHA. They surveyed 264 social workers and social work students employed at large urban hospitals known to treat sizeable numbers of PLWHA. While most respondents were well informed about the epidemic and demonstrated compassion for PLWHA, the authors found some resistance to working with this population. 60% of respondents reported they would be not very likely or not at all likely to work with PLWHA. Although most participants (91%) stated they would not refuse a case because of the client's serostatus, less than half (45%) expressed a current interest in working with PLWHA (Wiener & Siegel, 1990). When asked what might help them feel more at ease in working with PLWHA, respondents replied that more training about the virus and information about avoiding transmission; only 10% indicated that nothing would make them more comfortable (Wiener & Siegel, 1990). Some respondents shared that they viewed work with PLWHA to be emotionally exhausting, time and resource intensive, depressing, and potentially lethal (Wiener & Siegel, 1990).

Silberman (1991) researched the cognitive and affective demands experienced by MSW students (*n*=240) who worked with PLWHA during their practicum[7] education. 37%

of students reported they lacked adequate knowledge about resources in the community, while 34% were concerned about how to address their clients' feelings of distress and anger. These students were open to seeking support; 75% sought guidance from their practicum supervisor and 64% received informal supports from school faculty and other professionals in their placement. Students overwhelmingly (69%) recommended that future social work students should be placed with organizations that serve PLWHA. Respondents made several suggestions for educators, including: more education about transmission, resources, and social policy; confronting biases in faculty and other students against sexual minorities and IDU; specific courses about the needs of those populations; opportunities for students to explore their fears about death and their own mortality; and more individual and group supervision in their placements. (Silberman, 1991).

Frontline social workers and other helping professionals practicing during the worst days of the epidemic had to confront their own fears while constantly exposed to suffering and death. Martin (1988) notes "[t]he catastrophic experience of being sick with AIDS cannot be underestimated. Physical, emotional, and social hardships wrought by this disease are tremendous and taxing" (p. 1). Paradis (2003) describes a "culture of bereavement" (p. 479) where helpers and clients shared experiences of overwhelming grief and loss. Many social workers and other professionals shared identities with those most affected by the epidemic; several were living with HIV while working with PLWHA. Morin and Batchelor (1984) describe the challenges gay professionals working with PLWHA experienced:

> The psychological problems facing gay professionals who are dealing with AIDS are immensely complex. Many will over-identify with people with AIDS and push themselves too hard. Certainly, some who are confronted with AIDS patients

tend to resurface their own fears of AIDS and may become part of the "worried well". Others have special fears of contagion. The many gay practitioners who are not self-identified are faced with fears of backlash if it comes out that they are homosexual, and the anxiety over possible job loss and status, merely on the basis of being identified as gay, can be overwhelming. (p. 9)

McKusick (1988) explores the impact of HIV on therapist and client during the height of the AIDS crisis. He observes that countertransference reactions on the part of the therapist could be placed in three categories: anxieties around death and dying; concerns pertaining to intimacy and sexuality; and notions about caretaking and being taken care of. McKusick, who died from AIDS-related complications in 1993 (GLBT Historical Society, n.d.), notes how therapists need to address their own feelings of helplessness while serving their dying clients. He provides the example of a therapist living with HIV working with a PLWHA client. The work was complicated by the client's insistence that the therapist looked and talked like the client's deceased father. The client frequently asked about the therapist's serostatus. Eventually, the therapist disclosed that he was living with HIV, triggering feelings of loss in the client. The desire to assist his client was closely associated to the therapist's fears about his own mortality. McKusick urges therapists to develop an "inner ear" to assess their own countertransference prior to their work with PLWHA (McKusick, 1988).

Barret (1997) chronicles his experience with a client living with HIV who was rejected by his family and had few friends. As his client was dying, Barret frequently visited him in the hospital and contacted the client's treatment team. Barret was present for his client's final moments while holding his hand. Barret arranged the client's funeral and spoke at the gravesite. These actions seemed to go against the norms of the therapeutic relationship—“[w]hat I had done was ‘bend the frame’, maybe even twist the frame completely out of shape” (Barret, 1997, p. 44). As he addressed his countertransference, he understood the work demanded relational engagement and awareness of how his own issues might complicate the care of the client. Barret concludes that through suffering, he became more present for the client.

The emotional, physical, and occupational burdens experienced by social workers and other helpers during the height of the epidemic could be classified into three categories: general work stressors; stressors related to HIV/AIDS; and personal stressors (Ross, 1993). To address potential burnout—a state of emotional exhaustion and depersonalization—social workers were advised to adopt a holistic and multidimensional approach to stress reduction. Ross (1993) suggests that a model to reduce burnout would address five dimensions: cognitive (increased knowledge about the virus); emotional (opportunities to receive support from colleagues; breaks from regular duties); social (morale building events and involvement with social networks); spiritual-philosophical (evaluation of feelings regarding illness and mortality); and physical (exercise, yoga, balanced diet).

Social Work in the ART Era

As HIV transformed into a chronic and manageable condition, social workers encountered new challenges and opportunities. The demographics of the epidemic changed; the virus was increasingly affecting people of color, women, older adults, and those residing in the U.S. South (Kaplan et al., 2004). Evidence-based intervention models developed in the first years of the epidemic were not always grounded in the experiences and needs of these emerging sub-populations of PLWHA (Wheeler, 2007). Improved life expectancy and developments such as rapid HIV testing meant that social work with PLWHA could move out of hospitals and infectious disease clinics to more community-based settings (Linsk, 2011; Strug et al., 2002). The most monumental change was an increased emphasis on behavior change among PLWHA, especially concerning medication adherence. The optimism about new treatments was tempered by the reality that not every PLWHA responded to medications; furthermore, these regimens required personal commitment and consistent access to pills (Lowth et al., 1999). Ka'opua and Linsk (2013) describe the psychosocial challenges that PLWHA encounter with adherence, including: integrating complex regimens into daily life; maintaining motivation to take medications for indefinite periods of time; coping with possible side effects; dealing with stigma related to taking HIV medications; and utilizing social supports and spiritual resources to sustain quality of life. Social workers utilized interventions designed to increase medication uptake, including motivational interviewing, specialized adherence counselors, and integration of medication adherence into substance use treatment (Bass et al., 2013; Cooperman et al., 2013; Cooperman & Arnsten, 2005; Scheid, 2013). However, some social workers and other providers expressed concern that their work was too heavily focused on compliance rather than supporting the choices and self-determination of their clients (Lowth et al., 1999). Clients who saw no improvement in their health after adopting ART were sometimes assumed to be non-adherent and held responsible for treatment failure (Lowth et al., 1999). But adherence is not just a matter of getting drugs into bodies, as ACT UP memorably put it; there are a host of complex psychosocial issues that social workers and other providers were now charged with addressing (Auerbach & Hoppe, 2015; Ka'opna & Linsk, 2013).

Medication adherence was not the only social work challenge in the ART era of the HIV epidemic. Cain (2002) draws upon his studies of ASOs in Canada and addresses conflicts that negatively impacted the functioning of these agencies. Issues of identity and community caused schisms within ASOs; White gay male leaders were often seen to discount the concerns of others, especially women and racial minorities. Additionally, the professionalization of ASOs minimized the voices and experiences of PLWHA; some PLWHA felt that ASOs were more concerned with political agendas (such as addressing sexism, racism, and homophobia) than the immediate needs of clients. New organizations that focused on specific populations, such as women and people of color, were seen to be competing for scarce resources and unnecessarily duplicating services (Cain, 2002). Cain (2002) suggests that, as the demographic patterns of the epidemic changed, more tensions within and between ASOs were inevitable.

Poindexter (2007) describes the changing landscape of HIV social services as a "volatile surging sea" (p. 9). She notes that since PLWHA were living longer, ASOs were interacting with larger numbers of clients for longer periods of time, necessitating more dedicated staff and consistent sources of funding and other resources. Prolonged contacts meant that social work with PLWHA would require new directions, such as employment counseling, that would have been unthinkable in the earliest days of the epidemic. The increased professionalism and bureaucratization of services for PLWHA was seen as threatening the grassroots activist ethos that birthed ASOs, crowding out the volunteers who played a critical role at the onset of the epidemic and omitting the perspectives and input of PLWHA. Poindexter (2007) recognizes that as the epidemic's urgency diminishes among the general public, "HIV needs to be mainstreamed into existing social and health services, but not to the extent that ASOs are unable to sustain their unique contribution to community-based, consumer-centered, culturally competent care, prevention, and advocacy" (p. 23).

While ART provided hope for millions, an HIV diagnosis was still considered a life-altering event. Melendez (2010) notes that living with a chronic condition can negatively affect an individual's participation in social and community life. Social workers play a critical role in supporting PLWHA as they adjust to an illness requiring ongoing care and marked by stigma and discrimination. This work encompasses connecting clients to medical care, supporting them in navigating family and social relationships, exploring sexual health and harm reduction, and addressing co-occurring issues including mental health and substance use (Melendez, 2010). The continuum of care took place in more community-based and diffuse locales, including outpatient clinics (some of which were HIV-specific), home health care, skilled nursing facilities, assisted living facilities, and substance abuse/mental health treatment facilities, among others (Giddens, 2010). As PLWHA became integrated into community life, more social workers were required to develop knowledge of HIV and the capacity to meet the needs of clients living with the virus.

Social Work and HIV Today

Since the introduction of ART in the mid-1990s, scientists have made dramatic progress in designing drugs that are safer, more efficient, more effective, and less toxic than their predecessors (Maeda et al., 2019). However, medication adherence is still a barrier to viral suppression, especially for individuals who use substances (Krishnan et al., 2025; Tarfa et al., 2021; Whiteley et al., 2021). Mobile phone applications built to increase adherence have shown some promise in the short term, but long-term, sustained gains remain elusive (Knox et al., 2024; Martin et al., 2025; Mi et al., 2024; Roveta et al., 2025). Artificial intelligence (AI) and AI-based chatbots represent the next frontier in adherence science; however, concerns regarding client privacy and algorithmic bias remain salient (Ma et al., 2025; Olaboye et al., 2024; Sah et al., 2025). As new technologies develop, social workers and other professionals working with PLWHA will need to stay current with new approaches to this perennial dilemma.

Social workers assist clients with new methods of initiating and administering ART. Before 2017, standard medical practice was to delay ART uptake until baseline and drug resistance testing was completed (Dalal et al., 2023). Current protocols call for Rapid ART—the initiation of treatment on the same day (or within seven days) of the diagnosis, no matter the client's CD4 count (García-Deltoro, 2019; Mateo- Urdiales et al., 2019). However, Rapid ART is not yet standard practice due to lack of leadership and interdisciplinary collaboration, provider discomfort, and issues with expedited access to medication and benefits (Koester et al., 2022; Moran et al., 2023). Social work can facilitate this intervention and support clients in initiating and maintaining long-acting injectable ART which holds significant promise in HIV treatment, especially for individuals who may struggle with standard medication adherence (Scarsi & Swindells, 2021; Swindells et al., 2020). The rollout of long-acting ART been difficult for many reasons, including discrepancies between clients' desires and behaviors, risk of medication resistance, medical mistrust, insufficient infrastructure, and a lack of provider readiness to prescribe (Edwards et al., 2023; Fletcher et al., 2024). Consistent case management, flexible site administration, centralization of insurance authorization, and adherence monitoring are critical element of the success of long-acting ART interventions, all of which closely align with the roles and abilities of social workers (Fletcher et al., 2024).

The emergence of U=U (Undetectable=Untransmittable) represents another significant development in HIV care over the past decade. Calabrese and Mayer (2019) urge all providers to inform PLWHA that individuals who have achieved viral suppression cannot transmit HIV through sexual contact. They assert that this message could incentivize viral suppression and motivate treatment adherence. While there is increased awareness of U=U, negative attitudes and gaps in knowledge remain (Bor et al., 2021). In one study, over half (54.5%) of respondents did not know the meaning for U=U; individuals with a college degree or higher, more recent diagnosis, suboptimal ART adherence, and lack of communication with medical provider about the importance of undetectable viral loads, were less likely to understand U=U (Tadese et al., 2025). While Card and his colleagues (2022) found greater knowledge (72.6%) about U=U among their sample of 2681 participants recruited at Pride festivals across Canada, they acknowledge the importance of social positionality. They measured this concept using an index, giving each participant one point if they were (a) transgender, (b) a person of color, (c) Indigenous, (d) born abroad, (e) bisexual or straight, (f) not out, (g) struggling with money, (h) not college educated, (i) and not participating in LGBTQ2S+ organizations, queer pop-ups, or HIV advocacy organizations. With each additional point, a respondent was 21% less likely to know U=U (Card et al., 2022). Other studies suggest misunderstanding and skepticism about U=U, especially among those who are HIV-negative (Calabrese et al., 2024; Grace et al., 2021). In a recent survey of both PLWHA and HIV-negative individuals, nearly all participants (95.6%) were aware of U=U, but only 41.1% trusted the science. A greater percentage of PLWHA (66.0%) believed U=U compared to the negative/status unknown cohort (33.6%) (Calabrese et al., 2024).

Providers report challenges in discussing U=U, including concerns about "zero risk" messaging, a perceived lack of interest from clients, client mistrust and skepticism, and the need for more culturally appropriate resources (Grace et al., 2022). Social workers can leverage the message of U=U and address misperceptions that prevent the dissemination of this important intervention (Okamoto et al., 2024).

U=U is just one component of Treatment as Prevention (TasP), a public health policy to maximize engagement with HIV care, increase viral suppression, decrease HIV-related mortality, and prevent new infections (Lima et al., 2021; Montaner et al., 2025). This approach requires a status-neutral model of HIV care that proposes one treatment approach, regardless of an individual's serostatus (Myers et al., 2018). Individuals who test positive are introduced to and retained in HIV care, while those who test negative are offered pre-exposure prophylaxis (PrEP). While the paths diverge, they arrive at a common point (ART). Status-neutral approaches recognize that clients' health and social needs are not determined solely by their serostatus, but by a range of factors of which HIV is only one component (Pagkas-Bather et al., 2022). These interventions may reduce stigma and increase access for marginalized individuals, particularly people of color and transgender people (Driver et al., 2023; Gamarel et al., 2022; Knox et al., 2023). However, few status-neutral programs exist; social workers and other professionals must research and develop new ways to integrate this approach into community health care settings (Pagkas-Bather et al., 2022).

The success of biomedical interventions may obscure the enduring psychosocial needs of PLWHA. In their review of interventions to support Black men living with HIV, Goldhammer and colleagues (2021) find medication adherence was the most common outcome of interest. Notably missing were programs that minimize health barriers or address social determinants of health, such as housing. The World Health Organization (WHO) describes social determinants of health as "the conditions in which people are born, grow, work, live, and age, and the wider set of forces and systems shaping the conditions of daily life", including "economic policies and systems, development agendas, social norms, social policies and political systems" (World Health Organization, 2010). Medication alone will not end the epidemic without interventions that address root causes, such as systemic racism, homophobia, transphobia, disparities in healthcare access, poverty, food insecurity, housing instability, and criminal justice involvement (Bowleg et al., 2022; Brawner et al., 2022; Doshi et al., 2021; Menza et al., 2021). Individual-level behaviors, including condom use and ART adherence, do not sufficiently account for disproportionate HIV prevalence. Jeffries and Henny (2019) note that Black men, compared to White men, have lower odds of condomless sex, having multiple sex partners, and recent drug use, which are behaviors known to highly correlate with HIV infection. However, Black men tend to have lower educational attainment, lower income, and less health insurance coverage compared to White men, impacting access to health care. Interventions that fail to account for these factors will most likely fall short of their goals (Bowleg et al., 2022).

Today, social workers must move beyond interventions that focus exclusively on individualized behaviors. Rajabiun and colleagues (2025) had great success with a bundled intervention approach working with Black cisgender and transgender women living with HIV that combined elements of peer supports, trauma-informed behavioral health services led by Black women therapists, and improved linkage to medical care. Hammack and her team (2021) implemented innovative outreach strategies to engage difficult-to-reach populations and provide referrals for resources including transportation, job readiness, housing assistance, and insurance enrollment. Kuhns and colleagues (2021) examined structural factors that prevent transgender women of color from accessing HIV care. They found that clients who participate in services that address social determinants of heath (including housing referrals, employment training, and legal services) were more likely to remain in HIV care; however, only 48% of participants took advantage of these services (Kuhns et al., 2021). The authors note decreased involvement in the program over time, which may have been attributed to a lack of transgender care and/or transgender-affirming offerings. Social workers must continue to address structural barriers and inequities that harm clients' mental and physical wellbeing and exacerbate poor HIV outcomes (Endalamaw et al., 2024; Karram et al., 2024; Padilla et al., 2020).

Owens and colleagues (2023) explore the lived experiences of rural social workers who provide services to PLWHA. Participants were frustrated by constantly providing education about HIV and working to reduce stigma across multiple systems. They also reveal struggles with structural barriers, including housing shortages and inadequate health care,that make their work more onerous. Workers were pleasantly surprised and encouraged by the level of support they received from family and friends. To cope with job stressors, workers adopted strategies that emphasized the altruistic dimensions of their work and their impact on clients' lives (Owens et al., 2023).

Pakhomova and colleagues (2025) interviewed health care providers working with PLWHA to learn how they address noncompliance with treatment. Providers noted that relational approaches played an essential role in efforts to resume engagement. Often, this involved repairing trust that has been damaged by negative experiences with other providers. They describe the implementation of person-centered care where providers recognized the client's multiple needs, stressed trauma-informed approaches, and centered accessibility (Pakhomova et al., 2025). While this study explores the experiences of health care providers, the findings are relevant to the social work profession.

Labra and colleagues (2023) examine HIV knowledge and attitudes among social work students (n=674) in four countries. While respondents overall possesses positive attitudes about PLWHA, there were some concerns. Almost 1 out of 5 respondents (17.8%) disagreed that PLWHA should be able to work in professions dealing with the public, such as dentistry or hair styling (Labra et al., 2023). When asked whether PLWHA in their community should be allowed to fully participate in socio-cultural activities, a majority of respondents disagreed or had no opinion. A lack of knowledge may account for such attitudes. The researchers found that respondents had borderline low levels of HIV knowledge, with younger respondents possessing less knowledge than their older colleagues (Labra et al., 2023). These findings suggest that social work educators have a responsibility to incorporate HIV into their curricula to better prepare the next generation of social workers engaged with PLWHA.

The Early Career Social Worker Experience

This book explores the experiences of early career social workers engaged with PLWHA. The first years of professional practice represent a momentous turning point in the development of social workers, as they transition from the supportive confines of academic programs to more complex organizational settings where expectations and responsibilities increase. New practitioners often encounter intensive client needs and perceive a disconnect between theory and practice. Experiences during the formative years of social workers' development play a significant role in how they see themselves and their role in the profession, making the early career stage an important focus for scholars interested in identity formation, workforce sustainability, and the conditions under which social work practice occurs (Apgar & Dolan, 2023).

Stewart and Fielding (2022) note a range of terms in the book to define this professional cohort, including "social work graduates", "novice practitioners", and "newly qualified social workers". They prefer "early career social workers" because it more accurately captures the complexity of the liminal space in which practitioners assume new roles while developing the knowledge and skills necessary for effective and ethical practice. There is no agreement as to what constitutes "early career". Bates and colleagues (2010) investigate how early career social workers in their first year of practice perceived the effectiveness of their social work education. Glassburn (2020) explores the transition from MSW student to employee within 9 and 18 months post-graduation. McCullough and colleagues (2024) conducted a longitudinal study of early career social workers that examined learning over the first five years of practice. While "early career" has multiple operationalizations, research on this professional cohort underscores that this is a time focused on skill acquisition and identity formation within demanding and sometimes unstable practice environments (Apgar & Dolan, 2023).

One of the most widely studied aspects of early career social work is the transition from educational settings to professional practice. Several studies observe that early career social workers often feel unprepared for their new responsibilities. Tham and Lynch (2014) interviewed a small group (*n*=13) of Swedish social work students as they were about to graduate. Participants desired more exposure to clients and practitioners, as well as more instruction in practical skills. These students were mixed in their beliefs about their competence and preparation for practice. Four months after graduation, the authors (2019) re-interviewed the participants. These early career social workers felt insufficiently prepared for practice and struggled to manage difficult client conversations and interactions, including threats to their physical safety. They shared that they did not receive much onboarding or introduction to their organizations. Disappointment and disillusionment with their education, organizations, and the profession were common. The authors note that Swedish students receive significantly less practicum experience compared to social work programs in other countries, which could explain their perceptions regarding their preparedness.

Rentea and her colleagues (2025) explore how early career social workers in Romania understand their readiness for practice during their first three years post-graduation. Participants reported a mismatch between their classroom learning and the realities of practice and labored to apply broad theoretical frameworks to specific client situations. Limited agency resources, high employer expectations, and an absence of a formal transition from school to employment left these early career social workers feeling like they were, in the words of one participant, “thrown into a pit” (Rentea, et al., p. 162). Romania’s social work education infrastructure had to be rebuilt after the fall of the Communist regime in 1989; thus, it may be difficult to generalize this study to other countries. But similar findings have been replicated in different contexts. Glassburn (2020) interviewed early career social workers in the U.S. (n=27) within 9-18 months post-graduation. Most participants were generally satisfied with their education but felt unready for the emotional and practical challenges during the transition from school to employment. Participants were surprised by the variability in the quality and quantity of supervision and the early onset of burnout and compassion fatigue. Segev and colleagues (2022) conducted two focus groups in Israel, comprised of 11 early career social workers in total, in their first 18 months post-graduation. Participants were overwhelmed by their new roles and described a gap between their academic preparation and increased responsibilities. These challenges were heightened by difficult workplace conditions, substandard compensation, and a lack of supervision. The transition from student to early career social worker represents more than a change in title and status; it is a developmental period during which new practitioners must adapt to resource constraints and organizational demands while managing the emotional dimensions of social work.

Other studies offer a more optimistic appraisal of preparedness among early career social workers. Bates and colleagues (2010) conducted a mixed-methods study that explored the perceptions of new practitioners in their first year, as well as the perspectives of their supervisors. Most early career social workers agreed or strongly agreed they were well prepared in areas such as client communication, social work values, and responses to cultural differences. A substantial number felt less ready for tasks such as assessment, time management, and record keeping. Supervisors were generally more positive in their assessments of their supervisees' preparation for practice than the social workers themselves, suggesting a possible divide between perception and reality as to the readiness of early career social workers. Choi and colleagues (2015) examined six cohorts of early career social workers (*n*=246) between 9 and 15 months after graduation. Participants felt adequately or well prepared by their MSW programs to competently practice in their chosen field, in contrast to other studies. The book suggests that the transitional period may be experienced differently depending on cohorts, programs, and employment settings.

The challenges faced by social workers during the first phase of their careers are critical to professional socialization and identity formation. Moorhead (2019) describes professional identity as "the enactment of core features and norms of social work, particularly values, ethics, and purpose" (p. 207). She explores how early career social workers (*n*=17) experience professional identity within the first year of practice. The findings reveal three dimensions of the emerging social work identity: consolidation (ideas about the type of social worker they want to be); clarification (moving beyond the individual to determine what is unique about social work as a profession); and settling (am I worthy calling myself a social worker?). Participants were simultaneously managing the immediate duties of their positions and constructing a professional identity that extends beyond their current role. Afrouz and colleagues (2025) study how both early career social workers (up to 5 years post-graduation) and supervisors consider professional socialization, which they define as a "dynamic process through which new graduates develop their professional identity, integrating and adopting values, skills, and knowledge into practice" (p. 999). The early career social worker participants believed they did not yet belong to the profession, expressing self-doubt, uncertainty, and imposter syndrome. They also described a difficult balance between their personal selves and their nascent professional identity, trying to align their lived experiences with beliefs about professionalism. Early career social workers also adjusted to power relationships with clients and hierarchical systems within organizations that were uncomfortable and unfamiliar. Yao and Flynn (2025) draw upon a subset of their data (n=7) of early career social workers who claimed a social work identity within the first 6 months post-graduation. Participants stated their education and practicum experiences helped identify their strengths, preferences, and learning styles, which facilitated their fit within the profession. Assuming the mantle of "social worker" reinforced values and built confidence for decision-making. These studies demonstrate the early career period is a vital stage of professional socialization, during which social workers negotiate their professional identity while surviving the demands of practice.

Most research on early career social workers examines professional transition in more general terms and rarely attends to specific areas of practice, although some studies focus on child welfare practitioners in the beginning of their careers (Carpenter et al., 2015). To date, no research has been located that explores early career social workers engaged with PLWHA, nor how new social workers interpret complex social and political phenomena such as HIV during their first years in the profession. This study extends the book on both the epidemic and early career professional development, highlighting how social workers concurrently make meaning of HIV and find their place within the profession.

Conceptual Framework: The Socioecological Model

While individual-level interventions to promote behavior change have contributed to a decline in new infections, long-term success in eliminating HIV necessitates efforts that also address structural factors (Gupta et al., 2008; Jones et al., 2019; Rodriguez-Diaz et al., 2021). The socioecological model (SEM) is a frequently utilized framework that attends to the epidemic; a recent Google Scholar search of "socioecological model" and "HIV" resulted in approximately 18,300 results. SEM has been applied to the study of HIV testing behaviors in college-aged Black women (Dyson et al., 2018), PrEP uptake in sex workers (Ramos & Du Bois, 2024), barriers to couples' HIV testing for adolescent sexual minority men (Starks et al., 2021), and obstacles to viral suppression for transgender women living with HIV (Jain et al., 2023), to name just a few. The versatility of SEM is extensive; scholars have adopted SEM to study the prevention of sports-related deaths in high schools (Scarneo et al., 2019), explore maternal obesity (Hill, 2021), investigate gender inequities in computer science (Michell et al., 2018), and understand the challenges associated with young widowhood (Barros-Lane et al., 2024). This section provides an overview of the history and theoretical underpinnings of SEM with particular emphasis on its relevance to social work practice. Complementing SEM, a life course lens is introduced that adds a temporal dimension to the framework. Attention then turns to the use of SEM to study the experiences of helping professionals. Finally, the conceptual framework guiding this research project, which is informed by SEM, is presented.

History of the Socioecological Model

Given social work's historical interest in addressing both individual concerns and environmental factors, SEM is a particularly appropriate framework. At the 1901 National Conference of Charities and Corrections in Washington, D.C., there was a presentation of a diagram that visualized the sources of power and resources available to clients and their social workers. This diagram consisted of six concentric circles, labeled: family forces; personal forces; neighborhood forces; civic forces; private charitable forces; and public relief forces (*Cycle of Success: Librarian Finds Century-Old Line Drawing in Digital Library*, 2017). This visual tool demonstrated a comprehensive portrayal of the client's presenting issue, moving beyond individual concerns to address social and systemic factors; in this sense, it may be considered the precursor to SEM. The circle diagram, well known to social work historians was often attributed to Mary Richmond, a pioneering social worker and scholar. However, the diagram does not appear in *Social Diagnosis* (1917) or any of her other published works. She was one of the earliest social workers to elucidate a theory of practice that merged individual and environmental factors while addressing social concerns such as poverty and family discord:

> Individual differences must be reckoned with in every field of endeavor, but the theory of the wider self, though it has of course other implications, seems to lie at the base of social case work. We have seen how slowly such work has abandoned its few general classifications and tried instead to consider the whole man. Even more slowly is it realizing that the mind of man (and in a very sense

the mind *is* the man) can be described as the sum of his social relationships. (Richmond, 1917, p. 368)

Richmond's approach to social casework involves a diagnostic process where social workers collected information from multiple sources, including clients, family members, neighbors, employers, medical providers, and public officials. She acknowledges that as new social problems were introduced, new kinds of social work were required. For instance, with the introduction of laws restricting child labor, social workers were charged with new tasks, including verifying children's ages and assisting families looking for ways to compensate for the lost wages of the child (Richmond, 1917). Richmond asserts that social work that does not address the many facets of clients' lives was doomed to fail:

> There is, in fact, more resemblance than either would admit between the mental habits of the case worker who contentedly treats one individual after another, one family after another, without giving a thought to the civic and industrial conditions that hedge them about, and the mental health of the reformer who is sure that the adoption of his particular reform will render all social case work unnecessary. Both ignore the complexity, the great diversity, of the materials with which they are attempting to deal (Richmond, 1917, p. 367)

Richmond's ideas have played a foundational role in the development of modern social work practice (Agnew, 2004; Branco, 2018).

Psychologist Kurt Lewin's field theory influenced the development of the socioecological model. Lewin (1943) describes field theory as a method of analyzing causal relations and building scientific constructs. He believes that an individual's behavior is a function of both personal attributes and environmental factors. The individual resides in a "life space" consisting of the individual and their surrounding environment. Lewin (1943) introduces "psychological ecology" to describe the study of how individuals perceive, interpret, and are influenced by their life space. This approach emphasizes the totality of an individual's situation and encourages researchers to examine individuals and groups in relation to the internal and external forces that affect their experiences (Burnes & Bargal, 2017). Field theory was influenced by Gestalt psychology, which focuses the "here and now" of the individual; Lewin was less interested in past events or future possibilities (Burnes & Cooke, 2013). His pursuit of mathematical rigor and a highly complex topological model of the life space may have resulted in a decline of field theory, but his ideas remain prominent across many disciplines (Hinshelwood, 2018; Livneh et al., 2014; von Fircks, 2025).

Urie Bronfenbrenner, a developmental psychologist, is often credited as the founder of ecological systems theory. However, his ideas were partially inspired by the work of Roger Barker (1963, 1965), a psychologist who pioneered the field of ecological psychology. Barker, who worked with Lewin, concentrates on what he calls behavior settings—the physical locations where behaviors take place, such as schools or clubs. Several of Barker's studies are cited in Bronfenbrenner's most famous work, *The Ecology of Human Development* (1979). Bronfenbrenner refers to Lewin's formula describing behavior as a function of the person and environment.

One would therefore expect psychology, defined as the science of behavior, to give substantial if not equal emphasis to both elements on the independent side of the equation, to investigate the person *and* the environment, with special attention to the interaction between the two. What we find in practice, however, is a marked asymmetry, a hypertrophy of theory and research focusing on the properties of the person and only the most rudimentary conception and characterization of the environment in which the person in found. (Bronfenbrenner, 1979, p. 16)

Bronfenbrenner decries the state of developmental psychology and argues that the concept of environment was constraining, consisting only of a microsystem, defined as "a pattern of activities, roles, and interpersonal relations experienced by the developing person in a given setting with particular physical and material characteristics" (Bronfenbrenner, 1979, p. 22). Experiments limited in scope, divorced from the real-life contexts in which individuals reside, transformed his field into "*the science of the strange behavior of children in strange situations with strange adults for the briefest possible periods of time*" (Bronfenbrenner, 1979, p. 19, italics in original). To address the imbalance between person and environment, Bronfenbrenner (1979) proposes the ecology of human development, which he describes as the study of accommodation "between an active, growing human being and the changing properties of the immediate settings in which the developing person lives, as this process is affected by relations between these settings, and by the larger contexts in which the settings are embedded" (p. 21). In other words, there is a bidirectional relationship between the person and their environments that is defined by reciprocity—multiple factors influence and are influenced by other factors. These factors operate across the multiple systems in which individuals are situated. In addition to the microsystem, Bronfenbrenner (1979) describes the mesosystem (the interrelations among settings within the microsystem), exosystem (settings that do not involve the developing person directly, but in which events occur that affect or are affected by the developing person), and macrosystem (culture, beliefs systems, and ideology that underlie the other systems). Bronfenbrenner (1986) added the chronosystem, which highlights the role of time, life transitions, and historical events, to this model. This ecological approach views human development as a process in which an individual engages in activities that reveal, sustain, and restructure the environments in which they reside.

> Thus in the perceptual sphere the question becomes to what extent the developing person's view of the world extends beyond the immediate situation to include a picture of other settings in which he has actively participated, the relations among these settings, the nature and influence of external contexts with which he has had no face-to-face contact, and, finally, the consistent patterns of social organization, belief systems, and lifestyle specific to his own and other cultures and subcultures. (Bronfenbrenner, 1979, p. 28)

The ecological orientation provides a framework to guide research and place emphasis on the meanings individuals attribute to their environments and the motivational character of said environments, or what Bronfenbrenner (1979) describes as "the primacy of the phenomenological over the real environment in steering behavior" (p. 24).

Ecological perspectives were largely embraced by social work academics and practitioners. Carel Germain, a professor of social work at the University of Connecticut, is often credited with the introduction of ecological theories to social work practice. In the same year that Bronfenbrenner published his work on ecological development, Germain (1979) released her textbook, *Social Work Practice: People and Environments*. In the introduction, she critiques general systems theories that dominated social work practice in the 1960s, finding them too abstract and unhelpful for the design and implementation of interventions. Ecological perspectives offered to clarify the nature and functioning of the environment and provide insight into the individual/environment relationship.

> The professional purpose of social work arises from a dual, simultaneous concern for the adaptive potential of people and the "nutritive" qualities of their environment. In an ecological view, practice is directed toward improving the transactions between people and environments in order to enhance adaptive capacities *and* improve environments for all who function within them. To carry out the professional purpose requires a set of environmental interventions and a set of interventions into the transactions between people and environments to complement the sets available for intervening in coping patterns of people. (Germain, 1979, p. 8)

Germain asserts that adaptation lay at the heart of ecological social work theory. She believes that individuals are survival-oriented and, to ensure their continued existence, make continuous, change-oriented decisions to create goodness of fit between themselves and their environments (Germain & Bloom, 1999). Thus, the role of the social worker is to understand the factors that promote or hinder a client's adaptation and then intervene appropriately with a continuum of services that involve some or all the systems and individuals relevant to the client's situation. Germain's ideas continue to resonate in social work education and practice settings (Germain, 1973, 1978; Gitterman & Germain, 2008).

Greene (2017) identifies three reasons for the prominence of ecological theory in social work: it extends the profession's long-standing focus on both intrapsychic functioning and environmental conditions; conceptualizes the person and their environment as a unified system, avoiding artificial dichotomies; and draws upon multiple disciplines and theoretical traditions, including evolutionary biology, anthropology, Gestalt, and general systems, all of which are concerned with growth and change. Pardeck (1988) recognizes that social workers gravitate toward ecological approaches because they suggest that individual pathology is not the root cause of a client's presenting issues. Jack (2012) acknowledges the adaptability of ecological theory and application to a wide range of practice settings and client populations. The ecological perspective serves as one of social work's best known theoretical frameworks (Kemp et al., 2024; Mapson et al., 2021; Rogers, 2020).

There have been several critiques lodged against the use of ecological theory in social work practice. Brower (1988) believes that, though ecological models have conceptual appeal, they remain far too abstract for social workers to employ in practice. Ungar (2002) notes traditional ecological approaches position the social worker as an "expert" and do not always align with critical, feminist, and postmodern theories that recognize the role of power and oppression play in clients' presenting problems. He argues for newer ecological models, including Bookchin's social ecology and Naess' deep ecology, that are more adept at recognizing diversity and power dynamics between social worker and client (Ungar, 2002). Wakefield (1996a) argues social work does not require a "generic practice perspective in order to be a coherent, unified, and clinically effective profession" (p. 1). Methodically addressing and refuting seven arguments in favor of ecological theory in social work over the span of two articles (Wakefield, 1996a, 1996b), he asserts that the absence of explanatory power, "its lack of substantive assertions about the nature, strength, or changeability of specific causal processes" (1996a, p. 27), renders ecological theory ineffective. In social work's rush to atone for its past indifference to environment, Wakefield (1996b) worries the profession is losing its concern for the individual, that they were just one more system within a complex and ever-growingconstellationoffactors

Bronfenbrenner's ideas found favor in other disciplines that modified and extended his concepts. McLeroy and colleagues (1988), educators specializing in health promotion, offer the socioecological model (SEM) as a variation on Bronfenbrenner's ecological theory. Eschewing the systems topography, SEM focuses on five factors: individual-level (characteristics of the individual, including developmental history); interpersonal-level (formal and informal social networks, such as family and friends); organizational-level (social institutions including schools and work settings); community-level factors (relationships among organizations and institutions within certain boundaries); and public policy/social-level (including laws and policies) (McLeroy et al., 1988). The prefix "socio" stresses the significance of social networks and institutions to the model. Similar to an ecological approach, SEM addresses the reciprocity of interrelationships that support the factors of the model. However, while ecological approaches are more descriptive in nature, SEM provides more guidance in the design and implementation of interventions across multiple systems (Golden et al., 2015). As such, SEM advances ecological theory by translating its core principles into a structured framework for intervention and practice.

A Life Course Lens

While SEM offers a useful framework for studying the individual and environmental contexts where early career social workers engaged with PLWHA practice, it does not fully capture the temporal dimensions of personal and professional development. Life course theory affords a complementary lens that considers the significance of time and history. Together, SEM and life course theory allow for a more comprehensive understanding of how early career social workers engaged with PLWHA navigate their work, make meaning of the epidemic, and construct professional identities.

Life course theory considers how chronological age, relationships, common life transitions, and social change shape people's lives from birth to death (Hutchison, 2010). Elder and colleagues (2003) describe five paradigmatic principles in life course theory: life-span development (understanding developmental process requires a long-term perspective); agency (individuals make choices and compromises and are not passively acted upon by social forces); time and place (individuals are shaped by the historical times and places they experience); timing (when life events occur is often consequential); and linked lives (lives are lived interdependently and socio-historical influences are expressed through this network of shared relationships). Important concepts of life course theory include: cohorts (groups of individuals who experience social change at approximately same age/time); transitions (role and status changes that occur throughout the life course); trajectories (relatively stable long-term patterns of the life course); life events (discrete occurrences that may impact individuals); and turning points (major changes that alter trajectories) (Hutchison, 2019). While not as commonly utilized as SEM, life course theory has been applied in social work research in projects that investigate the effects of trauma and postmigration stress on the health of refugee women (Sangalang et al., 2022) and explore online incel (involuntary celibate) communities (Utterback, 2024). Life course theory can assist social workers looking to bridge "micro" and "macro" worlds and expand ideas of human development that extend beyond adolescence (Hutchison, 2005).

While SEM is the conceptual framework that supports this study, life course theory adds depth to how early career social workers experience clients, colleagues, organizations, and structural forces. Barrett and Barbee (2022) argue that life course theory is not just the study of what happened and when, but also the meanings that people impart to critical points in the life course. Taggart and colleagues (2020) assert that life course theory is useful in addressing the epidemic by offering a better understanding of the temporal significance of adolescence (a time when many individuals initiate sexual behaviors and/or substance use) and emerging adulthood (when individuals often first experience relationships, employment and parental responsibilities, and increased autonomy). Such insights allow researchers and practitioners to develop interventions that address life course factors that enhance susceptibility to HIV infection (Taggart et al., 2020). Papageorgiou and colleagues (2025) investigate the mental health and wellbeing of PLWHA in England through a life course lens. Employing the concept of biographical disruption, they found that younger PLWHA expressed sadness and shame that they would not experience life events similar to their peers, while older PLWHA lived through periods of grief and bereavement during the earliest years of the epidemic. But they also discovered that many PLWHA considered stressful moments as biographical reinforcements, or catalysts for personal motivation and growth. Steinberg (2020), also drawing upon the idea of biographical disruption, researches the emergence of chronic health conditions and their impact on identity formation for young adults. Her participants reported experiences of shaming and distancing, unable to participate in many of the activities that constitute sociocultural ideals of normative young adulthood. While Steinberg did not specifically address HIV, her work is salient to PLWHA in that she notes that conceptualizations of chronic conditions must take into account the role of timing.

A life course lens assists researchers studying how temporal context affects the work of social workers engaged with PLWHA. Villalba and colleagues (2025) explore how providers caring for older PLWHA frame aging with HIV. They describe how the timing of providers' commencement of practice with PLWHA explains their approach to client care. More experienced providers could articulate the monumental changes in the trajectory of HIV, both medically and socially. By contrast, less experienced providers only witnessed the era of the virus as chronic and manageable and have not observed patients dying in overwhelming numbers or seen the medical complications that come with AIDS. Providers were described as aging with their patients and experiencing the shifts in the epidemic alongside them. The introduction of ART was seen as a turning point in the epidemic. Providers noted that the medical aspect of treating PLWHA became more straightforward over time, changing their roles and interactions with patients (Villalba et al., 2025).

Apgar and Dolan (2023) adapt life course theory to conceptualize the career progression of post-master's social workers as a developmental process. They observe that social workers experience different stressors as they gain experience and become more accustomed to the challenges of their work. Early career social workers find themselves with fewer supports and resources, less clear expectations, and greater financial burdens due to student loan debt. Furthermore, early career social workers juggle pressures concerning licensure, lack of adequate supervision, and perceived disconnect between their MSW programs and the world of professional practice. This critical moment in the trajectories of social workers' professional lives requires developmentally attuned interventions, such as robust employment and supervisory support, to promote the growth and confidence of this cohort (Apgar & Dolan, 2023).

By incorporating a life course lens, this study situates early career social workers engaged with PLWHA as members of a distinct professional cohort practicing during a specific historical moment in the epidemic. This orientation allows for a more thorough examination of how timing and transitions inform the meanings participants ascribe to their work and the virus.

The Use of the Socioecological Model with Helping Professionals

Most studies relevant to social work practice that use ecological theories or SEM focus upon client populations that live with a particular psychosocial issue. However, these frameworks also support research that examines questions of how helping professionals make meaning of their work and interact with different systems on behalf of clients. Hill and colleagues (2023) apply SEM as their conceptual framework and explore the experiences and support needs of staff members employed at harm reduction programs. They identified eight themes across four levels of SEM but did not include policy/society-level factors. At the individual level, participants shared concerns about navigating physical environments and maintaining adequate self-care. Establishing relationships with clients and colleagues were themes developed at the interpersonal level. Focusing on the organizational level, participants discussed their positive and negative experiences with supervision, while at the community level, participants revealed the challenges of working with stigmatized populations in a stigmatized field and interacting with complex and inefficient systems (Hill et al., 2023). The authors note participants' narratives suggest key areas where organizations can deploy resources to prevent burnout and turnover, including additional training, increased compensation, and staff support groups.

Burnout and stress among social workers and other helping professionals have been the focus of several studies grounded in SEM and ecological systems theory. Habeger and colleagues (2022) offer recommendations for preventing burnout using a

SEM framework, including training interventions (individual-level), mentorship and peer relationship-building (interpersonal-level); improved supervisory support (organization-level), interdisciplinary collaboration (community-level), and advocacy for more funding and resources (policy/society-level). Chiarelli-Helminiak and colleagues (2022) use Bronfenbrenner's ecological systems theory to examine the factors that contribute to burnout among social work educators. At the microsystem, educators shared personal self-care activities, role strain, and relationships (positive and negative) with students and colleagues. Educators disclosed that, at the mesosystem, a major source of burnout was the inability to separate work matters from their personal lives. University leadership, university status, and accreditation stress were raised as contributors of burnout at the exosystem. At the macrosystem, educators emphasized lack of resources and frustration that social work values were not reflected at their institutions (Chiarelli-Helminiak et al., 2022). The researchers believe the ecological perspective allowed for a comprehensive understanding of the experiences of social work educators and their relationship to burnout (Chiarelli-Helminiak et al., 2022).

Lekganyane and Manganyi (2023) adopt an ecological systems approach in their study of the challenges of social workers employed in community-based care organizations for PLWHA in South Africa. They note the success of social work on behalf of PLWHA relies upon both individual change behaviors and programs that address poverty and inequality; therefore, researchers need an ecological systems approach (Lekganyane & Manganyi, 2023). The researchers described five themes implicated at all levels of the ecological system: managing psychosocial issues of clients, such as fear of disclosure; managing clients who refuse services; managing the socio-economic needs of clients, including unemployment and food insecurity; 4) minimal resources, including lack of transportation and inaccessible service locations; and 5) difficulties in implementing community-based interventions (Lekganyane & Manganyi, 2023). The authors state these barriers are best understood as a broad reflection of society, and thus resources, interventions, and trainings for social workers require the multisystem perspectives offered by ecological theories.

Ecological approaches, including SEM, have advanced research, fostered resilience, and supported social justice advocacy. de Lisser and colleagues (2024) developed their Social Ecology of Burnout model to study nurse practitioner burnout, highlighting that burnout is not an individual issue but a problem created by inattentive systems. Newell (2020) created an ecological systems framework for holistic self-care for social workers, situating resilience as a multifaceted process of well-being across different domains. Pickover and her colleagues (2020) offer an ecological framework to assist behavioral health professionals in thinking constructively how to integrate social justice advocacy into public health care systems. Extending ecological models to advocacy requires professionals to position themselves as actors within systems that have reciprocal effects and recognize that advocacy can be pursued within multiple systems, both working with and for clients (Pickover et al., 2020).

The Socioecological Model for Early Career Social Workers Engaged with PLWHA

A modified socioecological model (SEM) relevant to the experiences of early career social workers engaged with PLWHA is presented as the conceptual framework informing this book (see Figure 1). Many depictions of SEMs use nested concentric circle designs, starting with individual-level characteristics and then radiating outward to reflect expanding spheres of influence, from the interpersonal level to the level of policy and society. Such models are intended to demonstrate interdependence and interaction, suggesting that action at any one level ripples throughout the model and affects the other levels. There are limitations to such visual representations. Traditional illustrations of SEM suggest a "levels only" approach that minimizes interactions between different factors and focuses solely on the individual and/or interpersonal factors to the exclusion of other factors (Golden et al., 2015; Golden & Earp, 2012; Richard et al., 2011). Visual graphics inadequately convey the dynamic nature of socioecological theories (Luke & Stamatakis, 2012).

The proposed SEM adopts the elements of socioecological theory but advances a different way of thinking about how these factors impact the social worker engaged with PLWHA. The five groups of factors surround the social worker, eschewing a concentric approach that exclusively focuses on levels. The dotted lines in the model indicate movement and interactions between the groups of factors. The dynamism of this model conveys an attention to temporal forces; interactions occur across both time and place. The model represents the social worker as the nucleus of an atom, with the five factors as circling electrons. The social worker engaged with PLWHA may be surrounded by all or some of the factors simultaneously. At times, the factors collide and create conflicts that require social workers to engage with multiple dimensions of the model. Learning how to practice in a socioecological manner is a significant task in the social worker's professional development. The five groups of factors include:

- Personal: Factors that concentrate on the personal characteristics of the social worker, including their backgrounds, social work education experiences, knowledge of HIV and PLWHA, self-care strategies, and the individual impact of their work.
- Interpersonal: These factors center on the relationship and engagement between the social worker and client, looking at the client's HIV care, strengths and challenges of the client, the role of HIV in the lives of clients, and the social worker's use of self-disclosure with clients.
- Organizational: These factors encompass systems, policies, and interactions within the social worker's employment and/or practicum

setting. Important factors of note include intra-organizational collaboration, experiences with supervisions, job responsibilities and satisfaction, and the organizational response to current events.

- Community: Community factors address broader social and cultural contexts that shape attitudes toward HIV, looking at how the social workers makes sense of HIV stigma, intersectional stigma, and acts of discrimination. Community factors also include the social worker's collaboration with outside organizations.
- Policy/Societal: These factors involve laws, policies, and current events that impact social worker practice. Client and social worker responses to current events, questions about the relevance of HIV and the continued need for HIV-specific services, social worker experiences with larger systems, and thoughts about the future of social work with PLWHA are some of the factors in this group.

In Chapters 4 through 8, I explore each domain in detail and discuss how early career social workers engaged with PLWHA think and practice socioecologically. Each chapter stresses the porous nature of the boundaries between the factors, which interact holistically and remain in dialogue with each other. In Chapter 9, I synthesize the findings and discuss how early career social workers engaged with PLWHA make meaning of their personal and professional experiences, understand HIV, and become social workers.

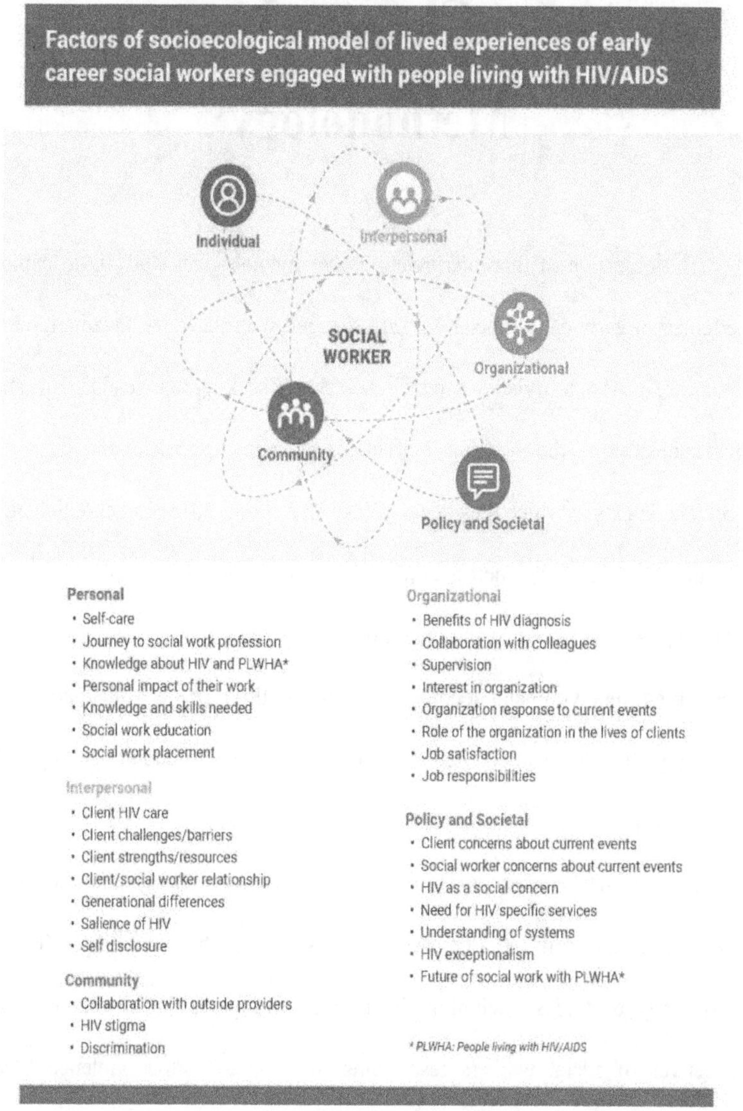

Figure 1: Factors of Socioecological Model of Lived Experiences of Early Career Social Workers Engaged with People Living with HIV/AIDS

Chapter 3
Methodology

The objective of this interpretative phenomenological study is to explore the experiences of early career social workers engaged with PLWHA. Qualitative research methods are most appropriate when the researcher is seeking to investigate questions of human subjectivity—the meanings individuals attach to experiences and life events and the social contexts in which they occur (Creswell & Poth, 2016; Engel & Schutt, 2016; Hammarberg et al., 2016). There are multiple approaches to qualitative inquiry, each with their own particular strengths and limitations (Creswell & Poth, 2016). For this study, I selected Interpretative Phenomenological Analysis (IPA). IPA is a qualitative research methodology that draws upon phenomenology, hermeneutics, and idiography (Miller et al., 2018; Smith & Fieldsend, 2021). While IPA was traditionally associated with psychology and health sciences (Houston & Mullan-Jensen, 2012), it has become more prevalent in social work research. Recent social work studies that utilized IPA cover a diverse array of topics, including the role of workplace social support from the perspectives of social workers responding to intimate partner violence (Brend & MacIntosh, 2021); the conceptualization of the child's voice in child protection practice (Williams & Parry, 2023); the transition to online teaching for social work educators (McCarthy et al., 2022); and the experiences of hospital social workers engaged with homeless clients (Winnett, 2022).

The aim of IPA is two-fold. First, researchers seek to provide rich and detailed descriptions of the personal meanings individuals ascribe to their lived experiences (Smith & Osborn, 2015). The concern is not with the phenomenon itself, but how the individual makes sense of the phenomenon under investigation (Eatough & Smith, 2017). IPA requires thorough examinations of personal perceptions, rather than objective reports (Smith & Fieldsend, 2021).

Second, IPA departs from traditional phenomenology in its embrace of hermeneutics, the study of interpretation. Rather than focusing on one individual's experience of a phenomenon, IPA examines the perceptions of a group of people, each of whom has had their own encounter with the phenomenon at the center of the inquiry. IPA attempts to understand the commonalities that exists among multiple experiences, as well as points of divergence (Miller et al., 2018). Researchers must consider how social structures, settings, and institutions impact an individual's meaning-making (Houston & Mullan-Jensen, 2012). IPA involves what Smith and Fieldsend (2021) describe as a "double hermeneutic": "[t]he participants are trying to make sense of their world; the researcher is trying to make sense of the participants trying to make sense of their world." (p. 53). The IPA researcher enters the world of the participant rather than merely investigating it (Eatough & Smith, 2017).

A defining feature of IPA is its commitment to idiographic research. Idiography prioritizes in-depth examination of individual cases, in contrast to nomothetic approaches that seek generalizable patterns across larger samples (Eatough & Smith, 2017; Miller et al., 2018). IPA focuses on in-depth analysis of each individual case prior to looking for patterns of convergence and divergence (Miller et al., 2018). Each participant is analyzed in detail, enabling the researcher to develop a nuanced understanding of their life experiences (Eatough & Smith, 2017).

Reflexivity Statement

A reflexivity statement allows the researcher to contemplate how their identities, experiences, values, and belief systems impact their methodology from the initial problem formulation to the final dissemination of the findings (Ide & Beddoe, 2024; Jamieson et al., 2023). Lazard and McAvoy (2020) assert the reflexive process is based upon two broad questions: "what is the research process and how am I influencing it?" (p. 167). Reflexivity is contrasted with reflection, which is more retrospective in nature and focused on what was missed or ignored during completed research (Jamieson et al., 2023). The research process is positioned as co-constructed through the dynamic interactions between the researcher and participants, with ongoing analysis and interpretation essential to a thorough account of the work (Sibbald et al., 2024). Scholars bemoan reflexivity statements that amount to little more than perfunctory lists of the researcher's positionalities without true examples of reflexivity (Sibbald et al., 2024). While some discussion of positionality is necessary to offer context for the researcher's reflexive practice[8], statements focused solely on the individual researcher neglect the larger social, cultural, and historical forces that shape the research process. I begin my reflexivity statement with an acknowledgement of my identities and experiences. Next, I consider the role of my background and beliefs, as well as historical and cultural forces that influenced my approach. Finally, I describe the steps I took throughout my research to engage in reflexive practice.

In December 2003, two doctors entered my hospital room. The older physician silently took my hand while his younger companion stood behind him, looking forlorn and anxious. The news was not surprising; I was diagnosed as HIV+. As a child of the 1980s, HIV/AIDS was a bogeyman unlike any other. The virus meant only one thing—death. And not just any death, but a shameful and sickening wasting away to nothing. Those afflicted with HIV were considered society's worst deviants—libertine gays, wretched addicts, and menacing immigrants. Growing up, I received scant sex education, and certainly no useful information about HIV. My beliefs about HIV developed during a time when fear, disgust, and ignorance dominated public discourse.

When I was diagnosed, there had already been important shifts in perceptions of HIV. New medications introduced in the mid-1990s brought hope to millions. HIV could now be treated and managed similarly to other chronic illnesses. As a gay male in my early thirties, I knew that outcomes for PLWHA were improving, but I could not escape the nagging thought that HIV was my destiny. For me, being gay meant that, at some point, I would become infected by this monster. Trying to navigate relationships and sex, in a world not always friendly to queer people, was difficult enough without worrying whether an intimate moment would prove ruinous.

HIV is a very manageable condition until it is not. As an educated White man raised with considerable economic advantages, my path to treatment was comparatively easy. When life was good, taking care of my HIV meant popping some pills throughout the day (and in later years, just one a day). However, at various times since my diagnosis, untreated substance use and mental illness robbed me of the ability to consistently adhere to my medications. The unchecked virus devastated and depleted my immune system and left me vulnerable to opportunistic infections that nearly resulted in death on more than one occasion. Over the past several years, I have taken charge of my health and manage my HIV well. Social workers and other helping professionals were instrumental in pulling me out of the abyss through counseling and medical assistance. I have a debt of gratitude, for which I hope this project offers some form of recompense. I disclose my history and identities not as a confession (Shelton, 2025), but as a window into how I see myself and my research. I note my positionalities and experiences do not serve as a "source of epistemic privilege" (Sibbald et al., 2024, p. 4). I do not hold myself out as a representative or stereotype of PLWHA. I strive to share my truth but claim no ownership of any universal Truth.

My interest in HIV as a topic of research began during my first social work job after graduating with my master's degree. In this role, I worked with GBT individuals at risk of substance use and HIV. In the early 2010s, I met a man in his early twenties who was recently diagnosed with HIV. He asked me whether he should tell his parents. I replied that since his parents were roughly my contemporaries, their ideas about the virus probably emerged at a time when famous people like Rock Hudson and Arthur Ashe were dying of AIDS, but that a lot had changed since those days. The young man looked at me with a quizzical stare, and I understood he had no idea who these people were or what I was talking about. It dawned upon me that his attitudes and beliefs about the virus were vastly different than mine because we each came of age during different eras of the epidemic. This encounter left me to wonder how my experiences and generational perspectives influenced my social work approach with PLWHA, and what this might mean for social work practice more generally.

As the worst years of the epidemic recede from public consciousness, I worry people have forgotten about HIV and PLWHA. Perhaps I will be forgotten as well. I see my research as a response to a collective amnesia. One of the great joys of my research has been meeting and talking with social workers doing amazing work with PLWHA. At a time when hope seems to be in short supply, I am comforted to know that people still care about the virus and those living with it.

My research was also impacted by my experiences in the classroom. I have taught social work at the graduate level since 2021, first as a part-time adjunct and now as a full-time instructor. While many of my students enjoy meaningful placements, I learned about deficiencies in their practicums, including inadequate supervision and learning opportunities. I am concerned about the readiness of new social workers to address professional challenges. My research is an opportunity for me to learn from early career social workers about their educational and work experiences. The stories shared by participants have provided me perspectives about the joys and frustrations of social work with PLWHA that I hope will translate into lessons that can support and advance social work education.

The memoranda drafted throughout the research process were essential to my reflexive approach. I obsessed whether this project was worthy of the time and effort. Did anyone really care about HIV? Do PLWHA still matter? My doubts, intensified by initial struggles with participant recruitment, were a dark cloud over my head. The first participant interview dispelled my worries. After years of study, reading, and writing, I was finally face-to-face (over a computer screen) with a live human being. That interview confirmed some ideas and challenged others. As the interviews continued, memo writing allowed me to voice my excitement, work through lingering concerns, and explore new lines of inquiry. One of the most consequential examples of reflexivity took place in February 2025. I drafted my initial interview guide in May 2024 and made some adjustments before the commencement of interviews in December 2024. The inauguration of Donald Trump in January 2025 altered the trajectory of my research.

Participants revealed their fears, anger, and uncertainty about the administration and the potential impact on client care and their own livelihoods. I shared their concerns. While I had always planned on asking about policy and politics, this topic felt more urgent. Observing how current events were impacting participants and their clients (and me), I explored this area in greater detail. I recognized through these interviews that lives and careers were at risk in the new political environment. By engaging in reflexive practice, I broadened the scope of my research and developed a sensitivity to the experiences of my participants that ultimately strengthened the research process.

Sampling and Recruitment

This study was approved by the Bryn Mawr College Institutional Review Board (IRB) (Protocol #24-060) on May 10, 2024. Subsequent amendments to the study protocol were approved on October 1, 2024, October 14, 2024, and February 14, 2025. IPA most often involves the use of purposive sampling techniques (Houston & Mullan-Jensen, 2012). Purposive sampling is a nonprobability method in which individuals are invited to participate in a study based on their experience with the phenomenon of interest (Brend & MacIntosh, 2021; Williams & Parry, 2023). Many IPA studies are conducted with relatively small sample sizes because of the in-depth, time-consuming idiographic analytic approach (Smith & Fieldsend, 2021). However, there are no established guidelines for determining an appropriate sample size. McCarthy and her colleagues (2022) interviewed 17 social work educators about their perspectives on transitioning to online classes from in-person education. By contrast, an IPA study of the experiences of undergraduate students who do not consume alcohol involved only 5 participants (Conroy & De Visser, 2014). Homogeneity is a defining consideration in sample selection, as participants are chosen for their shared likelihood of having encountered and made sense of the phenomenon of interest (Larkin et al., 2019).

In the initial IRB protocol, individuals were invited to participate in this research study if they met the following inclusion criteria: a) current MSW student or recent graduate (within 2 years of date of interview); b) who worked with at least 2 PLWHA during their practicum placement(s) over a period of at least three months; and c) resided and/or worked in a large Northeastern city and/or its surrounding counties. My first outreach efforts consisted of e-mails and telephone calls to directors of practicum education and other social work education administrators. Attached to the e-mails were a recruitment letter and flyer meant for wider distribution (see Appendices C and D). I also e-mailed and called social services organizations and medical providers engaged with PLWHA. However, despite vigorous efforts, this first recruitment wave was unsuccessful. After consultation with my Director of Work, I removed geography from the inclusion criteria. I resumed my recruitment efforts and broadened my reach. Using the Council on Social Work Education (CSWE) website, I obtained contact information for the directors of practicum education for 241 accredited MSW programs and sent e-mails with the recruitment materials attached. I also sent an email and materials to the mailing list of the LGBTQ Caucus of Social Work Students & Faculty (Q Caucus). I posted information about the study on a social media networking site (LinkedIn), which was shared by my colleagues within their networks. I also circled back to the schools and organizations I contacted during the first round of recruitment. Six participants were successfully recruited during this second wave.

Once again I met with my Director of Work, and we decided to further open the inclusion criteria. We amended the criteria to: a) current MSW students or early career social workers (received their MSW within 10 years of date of interview); b) who worked with at least 2 PLWHA for at least 3 months at their practicum and/or place of post-MSW employment; and c) worked and/or resided in a major Northeastern city and/or its surrounding counties. IRB approval for these changes was granted. I began my recruitment efforts anew, using similar methods as before. Not surprisingly, as the criteria expanded, I recruited more participants in a relatively short period of time. As the number of participants grew, I also used snowball sampling, whereby new participants are identified by preceding participants (Handcock & Gile, 2011; Parker et al., 2019). At the end of data collection, I completed 23 interviews. I excluded one interview because the participant did not meet the inclusion criteria (they had graduated with their MSW more than 10 years prior to the interview). The final sample size was 22. See Table 2 for information about the composition of the sample.

Table 2

Sociodemographic Characteristics of Study Participants (n=22)

Characteristic	*n*	%
Gender Identity		
Genderqueer/Non-Binary	9	40.9
Female	7	31.8
Male	6	27.3
Racial Identity		
White	16	69.6
Black	2	8.7
Hispanic	1	4.3
Hispanic/Middle Eastern	1	4.3
Other	1	4.3
White/Asian	1	4.3
Age Range		
20-29	7	31.8
30-39	12	54.5
40-49	2	8.7
50+	1	4.3
Years of Post-MSW Experience		
Current MSW Student [a]	5	22.7
<2 years post-MSW	7	31.8
<5 years post-MSW	4	18.2
<10 years post-MSW	6	27.3
Social Work Settings/Responsibilities (*n*=36) [b]		
Medical Case Management	17	47.2
Mental Health	8	22.2
Substance Abuse	5	13.9
Youth Services	2	5.6
Housing Case Management	2	5.6
Administration	1	2.8
Research/Evaluation	1	2.8

[a] All current MSW students stated they were to graduate in 2025.

[b] Some participants had more than one placement/employment working with PLWHA.

The sample is very diverse in terms of gender identity, with a substantial percentage of participants reporting a genderqueer or non-binary identity. While an overwhelming number of participants are White, approximately 30% of the sample identify as People of Color. The mean age of the sample is approximately 33 years old. Over half the sample are current MSW students or social workers with less than 2 years of post-MSW experience. Participants worked with PLWHA in a variety of settings; medical case management and mental health services were the most frequently mentioned roles.

Data Collection

The semi-structured interview is the most common form of data collection in IPA research (Miller et al., 2018; Smith & Fieldsend, 2021). This method allows for naturalistic conversation between researcher and participant while honoring the commitment to an idiographic process (Williams & Parry, 2023). After a book review, I drafted the initial interview guide. The guide was modified after the changes to the inclusion criteria and was approved by the IRB (see Appendix A). All interviews took place between December 2024 and April 2025.

Each participant was sent a consent form which they were asked to sign and return via e-mail prior to the interview (see Appendix B). Participants were asked to select a pseudonym that would be used in the dissemination of study findings. All interviews were conducted over Zoom; only the audio portion of the interview was recorded. Before each recording, I asked the participant if they had any questions or concerns. Once the recording began, I confirmed with the participant that they had read and signed the consent form and offered an opportunity for any questions about the consent form or the interview process. Demographic information was collected at the outset of the interview. Interviews ranged from 56 minutes to 92 minutes; the mean interview length was 72.3 minutes. Within 24 hours of each interview, I sent the participant a $35 gift card to the vendor of their choice as compensation for their time.

The audio file for each interview was uploaded to Cockatoo, an online transcription tool. A preliminary transcript was generated. I listened to the audio file while reviewing and revising the transcript. On a secure, password-protected, cloud-based storage service, I saved for each participant their consent form, interview transcript, receipt for gift card; and memorandum. These data will be retained for three years, in compliance with Bryn Mawr College IRB policy. The audio files of each interview have been deleted.

Data Analysis

The analytic focus of any IPA study lies in attending to participants' individuals experiences while interpreting those experiences within broader social and theoretical frameworks (Miller et al., 2018). Data analysis takes place in two phases. In the first phase, the researcher carefully details the experience of each participant. The second phase seeks to interpret experiences through discovery of convergences and divergences within and between the transcripts (Conroy & De Visser, 2014). McCarthy and colleagues (2022), drawing upon the work of Larkin, Flowers, and Smith (2021) detail six steps of analysis: reading and reviewing each transcript; coding each interview line-by-line; identifying emerging themes; examining connections between emerging themes; repeating this process with each interview, while recognizing pervasive themes across interviews; and linking between themes and creating concept maps and figures to make sense of the data.

My analysis began by carefully reading and re-reading each completed transcript. I drafted an analytic memo for each transcript summarizing the interview, offering my thoughts and feelings about the data and the interview process, identifying emerging themes and directions to explore, and outlining next steps in the data collection process. I uploaded all transcripts to Dedoose, a web-based platform designed for qualitative and mixed methods research. Dedoose is relatively simple and convenient to use and was a good choice for this project. Before starting my coding, I once again read each transcript. I did not begin my coding until all the interviews were completed. I randomly selected the order of transcripts and broke the sample down into small groups. For the first round of coding, I utilized *in vivo* coding. *In vivo* coding is an analytic technique whereby the researcher uses the participant's own words and phrases to capture their experiences (Rogers, 2023; Saldaña, 2021a). Saldaña (2021b) distinguishes between "lumpers" and "splitters". A lumper may use only one word or phrase to represent an entire excerpt, while a splitter goes line-by-line and divides the excerpt using multiple *in vivo* codes. I was in the latter category. Saldaña (2021b) notes that while the splitter may scrutinize the data, they can become overwhelmed by the sheer number of codes. This was my experience; despite my best efforts, I would up with hundreds of in vivo codes for each transcript. After finishing a group of five transcripts, I drafted an analytic memo discussing my process, describing interesting concepts from the data, and refining my coding approach. I repeated this process until completion of the first round. I was drowning in a sea of codes, but appreciated how this technique provided me familiarity with the data.

Before commencing the second round of coding, I re-read all the transcripts and reviewed the first-round *in vivo* codes and consulted my analytic memos and memos for each transcript. According to Saldaña (2021b), memo writing serves as an important method for generating codes and categories. Drawing upon my book review and emerging conceptual framework, I recognized important concepts and themes emerging. I developed new codes to reflect each participant's experiences with the five levels of SEM: individual, interpersonal, organizational, community, and policy/society. I turned to focused coding for the second round. Drawing upon the work of Charmaz (2006), focused coding is a streamlined analytic process through which the researcher refines and develops the most salient categories within the data (Onwuegbuzie et al., 2016; Saldaña, 2021b). I found this to be a more manageable process than the first round; however, I realized the benefits of intensive engagement with the data before commencing the second round. Using the categories and themes from the second round, I sketched a map to visualize what the data were showing. That map was refined and expanded and serves as the conceptual framework.

Rigor and Trustworthiness

Nizza and colleagues (2021) identify four key markers for assessing the quality of IPA research. First, good research should tell a compelling narrative built upon carefully selected extracts from the transcripts of participants. Second, there must be a vigorous experiential account that engages with the significance of what participants are reporting. Third, researchers must engage in a close analytic reading of participant quotes; words should not be left to speak for themselves. Finally, IPA studies take special care to attend to patterns of convergence and divergence within and between individual accounts. Throughout the research process, I have sought to meet these benchmarks through close, iterative engagement with the data and detailed reporting of the findings.

IPA researchers utilize different methods to enhance the trustworthiness of their work. Memos that record reactions to individual interviews help researchers concentrate on the participant experience rather than their own perspectives (McCarthy et al., 2022). I made extensive use of memos throughout the data collection and data analysis stages.

Consultation and debriefing with colleagues also ensure rigor in IPA studies (Brend & MacIntosh, 2021; Winnett, 2022). I met my Director of Work on a monthly basis during the data collection period and engaged in several discussions with colleagues who have worked with PLWHA. These conversations helped to address challenges and develop new ideas and lines of inquiry. Allowing participants an opportunity to review their transcripts can serve as a check on the researcher (McCarthy et al., 2022). All participants were asked at the end of the interview if they wanted to review their transcript and six participants stated that they wished to do so. No participants who were sent their transcript shared any concerns or objections.

Ethical Considerations

The NASW Code of Ethics (2021) calls upon social workers to maintain and promote high standards of practice and engage in research consistent with commonly accepted ethical principles. Throughout all stages of the research process, I have sought to align my work with the values of the profession. This project received IRB approval at the outset, as well as for all subsequent amendments. I explained to each participant their rights as a research subject, including the ability to stop the interview at any time and request their interview be deleted. I provided details about safeguarding the data and identities. Participants were fairly compensated for their time. In the dissemination of my findings, I omit specific identifying information about participants. However, it is possible that some readers may be familiar with the participants. Even when conducting research in large, well-populated areas, social work can seem surprisingly small. This is especially true given the nature of social work with PLWHA.

An ethical issue that arose during the research process was my prior knowledge of some of the participants. There were three participants that I had met before but with whom I did not have longstanding relationships. After consulting my Director of Work, we felt that my passing acquaintance with these individuals did not pose any ethical concerns. Two participants were former students of mine. I discussed this issue with my Director of Work. Given the absence of an ongoing power relationship and lack of contact since they were my students, their inclusion in the study was determined to be ethically appropriate. The IRB was notified of this issue.

Chapter 4

Individual-Level Experiences of Social Work Practice with PLWHA

At the individual level, the socioecological model emphasizes the personal characteristics and experiences that affect how social workers engage with PLWHA. These factors, including personal values, educational background, knowledge of HIV, and prior life experiences, directly influence how social workers perceive clients and manage the complexities of their practice. Understanding these individual-level factors is crucial because they create the foundation upon which interpersonal, organizational, and structural dynamics emerge, affecting both the quality of care afforded to PLWHA and the wellbeing of social workers. In this chapter, I examine the individual-level factors of the proposed socioecological model. Analysis of the data revealed seven themes: the journey to the social work profession; prior knowledge of HIV and PLWHA; experiences in social work education; practicum experiences; the knowledge and skills required to work with PLWHA; self-care practices and strategies; the personal impact of the work on the social worker.

Journey to the Social Work Profession

Individuals pursue social work for many reasons, including altruism, the desire for a sustaining career, and previous experiences with helping professionals

(Csikai & Rozensky, 1997; Petersén, 2024; Stevens et al., 2012). Some participants described how they were inspired by the values and history of the social work profession. Vanessa, a current MSW student who had previously received a Bachelor of Social Work (BSW) degree, discussed how a day at the library convinced her that social work was her destiny.

> I was leaning towards social work or education. I just always knew that I wanted to help people, but I never knew in what type of form I wanted to do so. It was a 50-50 choice for me, either social work or education. I chose social work, but it didn't really set in to me until I was like, I learned this very vividly. It was like, I was in the library, at 10:00 am, reading my readings, just my first semester into the social work program, undergrad. And I was reading about advocacy and how just like, I'm Jane Addams, and you know, the history of social work. And that's when a wave of emotions just hit me. And I started crying. I'm like, this is where I'm supposed to be. I've made the right choice and that was like the most clarity I've ever felt like ever and I was like maybe 19 or 20 at this time. So, this was a really weird feeling for me and ever since that day people have been laughing, people always looking at me crazy, crying at 10 in the morning reading…I'm happy with my choice and I really do believe that I was just guided in the right direction. And that's who I am now. (Vanessa)

For Vanessa, the story of Jane Addams and the history of social work resonated deeply. The values of the profession and its broad reach proved to be a good match for Vanessa's wish to help others. In a similar vein, August, a social worker with ten years of experience, explained how his introduction to social work as an undergraduate established his professional trajectory.

> I didn't know what social work was until going to college. I started off as a music performance major and hated it a lot. I completely fell out of love with music the moment I was required to spend four hours a day in a practice room. And I had some friends who were social work majors, and they told me I should enroll in a social work class that also would fulfill a gen ed requirement, and I did. And that professor was one of the most exciting, passionate people I've ever witnessed in a classroom. And the way she talked and embodied social work was just so amazing to me. And it felt, I felt just completely at home learning about human behavior theory, human development, and social justice, and specifically topics that impacted the queer community where I was excited to be in a community where we were actually talking about that and trying to find ways to pursue social justice with that community. (August)

August's alignment with the values of social justice and interest in working with queer communities positioned social work as a logical career choice. For Vanessa and August, exposure to the history and principles of the social work profession inspired turning points that reoriented their career trajectories and initiated the formation of social worker identities rooted in the social justice ideals and socioecological orientation of the profession.

Other participants described their journey to social work as a second career path illuminated by their involvement with social workers and other helping professionals. Bryan, a recent MSW graduate with less than two years' experience, was asked how they would describe their journey to the social work profession.

> Unexpected. Also very, it felt so right. I was a performer all of my life since I was a child. I love singing and acting, and I pursued that for most of my life. The pandemic happened and, you know, the industry was sort of put on pause indefinitely and it really made me question so much of what I was doing with my life. You know, my body was really exhausted as a dancer. I'd been in therapy myself since I was 19 and I just found it so life-changing, so helpful. Mental health and psychology had always been such a fascinating field for me, like I think that did go sort of hand in hand with performing, like just really very human-ish. And I was in therapy during the pandemic and I just, it like kind of
> just clicked, like I was, oh I want to do what you're doing, like my therapist, and it just inspired the path to apply back to school, and yeah, I'm really loving it. (Bryan)

Bryan's motives to become a social worker are a complex intersection of personal, physical, existential, and professional motivations that transpired during a historical moment that served as a "career shock" for many individuals who lost jobs or started new ones in the aftermath of the COVID-19 pandemic (Akkermans et al., 2020). COVID-19 was not merely an epidemiological event, but a social, economic, and political turning point that resulted in individuals and institutions re-assessing their priorities and practices (Purkey et al., 2022; Settersten Jr et al., 2020).

For other participants, the decision to become a social worker was more pragmatic. Dan, a social worker with more than five years post-MSW experience, was inspired by the profession's values and his belief that social work would be a quicker route to his ultimate goal.

> Yeah, I mean, I'll be honest, it was definitely a combo. I think part of me wants to say it's just for the values and the social justice component. That's definitely part of it. But I also think the reality of committing to like a five-year Psy.D. or something else, so the financial commitment, the time commitment, and I think this is one of those weird spaces where you can't know what it's like in the space until you've actually completed the degree. So, the idea that I was going to commit to a five-year degree with the possibility that I might not actually enjoy what I end up in. So, I think there was a balance of efficiency, but also the values of the work itself were appealing. (Dan)

For Simon, a social worker with almost ten years of experience, the versatility of the MSW degree was more appealing than other helping professions.

> My journey to social work, it's interesting. My journey in social work, it came, it actually originated as an interest in psychology, and I thought I would just be a counselor and, you know, follow that whole psychology route. However, after graduating from REDACTED with my BA in psych and a minor in sociology, I did some research and talked to people. And social work, I learned that it's a very broad degree. It's not just child welfare work, which tends to be the general gist of it. And then learning that it's just a more versatile degree, it's very broad, and you do so much more with it. So that's how I came into social work. (Simon)

While each journey is distinctive, the desire to serve others and establish a meaningful career is featured prominently throughout the stories of the participants.

Knowledge of HIV and PLWHA

Participants were asked to share their knowledge of HIV and familiarity with PLWHA prior to engaging with this population. According to one recent study, 52% of Americans feel knowledgeable about HIV, while 37% knew only a little about the virus. 10% had heard of HIV but did not know much about it, while 3% were not aware of HIV. In the past five years, there has been less comfort in having a neighbor (67% today vs. 71% in 2020) or co-worker (64% vs. 69%) living with HIV. This study found that Gen-Z individuals (approximately ages 14-29 in 2026) are the least knowledgeable about HIV; 37% of respondents in this generational cohort agreed that they feel knowledgeable about HIV (GLAAD, 2024).

Younger participants acknowledged they had little knowledge about HIV prior to working with PLWHA. The mean age for participants is 33 years old. This cohort of early career social workers (with some notable exceptions) has no memories or lived experiences of the worst years of the epidemic. This distance colors the worldview of participants. When asked what they knew about HIV before starting their first social work practicum, Bryan noted they came of age when the virus was considered a vague but still fearful memory.

> To be honest, like not much. And I think like, I, so I'm (early thirties), I did not grow up during the AIDS epidemic, but I definitely grew up very much like in the aftermath of, my mom very much was like, so scared for me, like always. And so I think that my knowledge of it was like, it is a scary disease that if you get it's like a death sentence, but that really started to change maybe in my late teens when I feel like you really started to hear about medications,

people not having any real issues as long as they're medicated. So that's definitely soothes a lot of my knowledge, I guess, I mean it soothes any fears. But in terms of other knowledge, I guess I just know that it compromises your immune system and so it essentially takes away your ability to fight infections. And so the littlest of any kind of virus or bacteria will be significantly more harmful. So that's my, that's, that felt like my basic understanding. (Bryan)

Growing up in the years after the introduction of ART, Bryan believed that HIV could be well managed but was still a "scary disease". They stated that as their understanding about HIV increased, anxieties about the virus were ameliorated. Research suggests that more knowledge about HIV may result in more favorable attitudes about PLWHA (Ferguson et al., 2023; Spence et al., 2022). Dan remarked that his rudimentary knowledge about HIV was supplemented by his friendships with queer individuals.

> I would share that I think what was learned in high school and other parts of my life was probably tempered by having queer friends who would date or have people they knew who would talk about like U equals U. I think I had one friend that comes to mind who had referenced experiences. I think I'd already had some exposure to this as an idea. I think devoid of some of that or devoid of having queer friends who talked to me about some of this, I think my understanding would have been really a bit more limited and probably problematic because it was just informed by probably a more outdated high school curriculum. (Dan)

Dan's lack of knowledge about HIV, outside of what he learned from his queer friends, may be explained in part by the fact that he identifies as straight. Since the onset of the epidemic, HIV has often been portrayed as a "gay issue" (Herek & Capitanio, 1999; Smit et al., 2012). Participants who identified as queer tended to have more prior knowledge and interest in HIV. Issa, a recent MSW graduate with less than two years' experience who identifies as queer, recalled how their previous work as a peer educator in high school prepared them for their first-year MSW placement working with PLWHA.

> I felt like I knew a lot from that peer education that I did in high school, because the first part of it was doing maybe like six months of weekly classes that went over all kinds of things, again, with sort of like an HIV/AIDS focus. I got the feeling at REDACTED that they were not sure how much I knew necessarily, which makes sense. And I was like, oh yeah, like I know what those things mean. (Issa)

Issa is a member of Gen-Z. Given their generational position, it would not be unusual for their practicum agency to be concerned whether they had prior knowledge of HIV.

Josh, a social worker with less than two years post-MSW experience, shared that their knowledge about HIV came from close connections with PLWHA. Josh was one of the oldest participants in the study. While they belong to the cohort of early career social workers, their personal experiences with PLWHA set them apart from most participants. Josh's first-year practicum was at a recovery home where they worked with many PLWHA; they are now a psychotherapist with two clients living with HIV.

I do not know as much as, like, someone who, like, maybe specializes in working with clients with HIV, or like, I'm not a virologist, I don't know. But I've worked with a lot of people who have HIV, like the people at the recovery house...half the people had HIV...sometimes gay sex, sometimes from a needle exchange. And I just, I've lived with a lot of people who have HIV and who, a lot of people who survived AIDS, like the peak of AIDS, like lost hundreds of friends. And so, I think I just, I just learned a lot about, you know, that experience, and that the need around it. So, I think I'm just somewhere in the middle of like, I'm not an expert, but I know way more than the average individual who only knows like the propaganda shit or the stuff that's on television about having HIV. (Josh)

Josh acknowledged the role of popular culture in shaping beliefs and attitudes about the epidemic. Media and popular culture have shaped discourses about HIV, both positively and negatively (Farrell, 2006; Hart, 2014; Johnson, 2013). August recalled how his first understanding of HIV came from a well-known musical.

I think the very first time in the media, because I was born in (early 1990s), so it was later than the center of the AIDS epidemic, but *Rent*, the musical, was honestly the first time I ever really remember being exposed to it in real life or pop culture. I think that's something that I wish just the high school, middle school sex ed would really talk about more is actually HIV and STI prevention and like the whole spectrum of prevention to care and like what that looks like. I think that's something that I'm talking to youth experiencing homelessness and even today, like they're not getting a really in-depth or even surface level education on HIV and STIs and don't feel like it's important until they're impacted by it, or they know somebody directly who's impacted by it. (August)

August noted that his age placed him outside of the worst years of the epidemic; this historical context helps explain his reliance on popular culture in the absence of any sort of comprehensive health education during secondary school. August also emphasized that, in his work in the HIV field, he has not observed much educational programming about the virus. This lack of attention may reinforce the perception that HIV is no longer a pressing concern.

Social Work Education

Participants were asked to share their classroom experiences in their MSW program, the presence of HIV in their curricula, and their opinions whether their classroom learning had adequately prepared them for social work practice post-graduation.

Experiences in the Classroom

Participants were decidedly mixed in their satisfaction with the classroom element of their social work education. Dan had an overall negative experience in his social work program, although he appreciated the learning he accomplished through his practicums.

> I wouldn't say I cared for it that much. Yeah, I mean, I've spoken to a variety of folks in other programs, and it sounds like it was a shared experience. But I think the school, on the front end, I think they advertised a certain experience that wasn't what I had. I had like a few classes that were decent. The majority were very mediocre. And yeah, I think the main thing I got out

> of it was the opportunity to be in internships where I had a lot of exposure. So I feel kind of conflicted about, you know, we're spending all this money to effectively volunteer our time in spaces that aren't really well monitored or tended to. But experientially, I think, like, I was really lucky to get really solid internships, which I think helped out for later on. (Dan)

T, a current MSW student who completed their second-year placement working with PLWHA, shared a similar frustration and identified a disconnect between the classroom and practicum learning.

> See, now you also did something that I'm very outspoken about, which is I think that the program that I'm in is really not great. And for so much of what I've been doing, it has been what I've learned at the clinic versus what I've learned in the classroom. And it has to do with the way the professors are teaching the class and the lack of structure they have when it comes to teaching their classes. There are quite a few teachers within the master's program here that I love and enjoy so much, and they have genuinely taught me so much. But there's also, on the same side, so many bad professors here who frequently go off on tangents about things unrelated to the coursework or literally, I don't even know what they're teaching half the time because it they're just saying words…But it frustrates me that there are so many things that could be so helpful, and like these classes could be so beneficial, but I'm not learning anything. (T)

Students can feel discouraged by what they perceive as discrepancies between learning in classroom and learning in practicum (Grady et al., 2020; Morris et al.,

2024). This gap can lead to further frustration once students enter the profession and report feeling unprepared for their job responsibilities (Tham & Lynch, 2019).

Other participants were more satisfied with the classroom element of their programs. Scott, a recent graduate with less than 2 years' post-MSW experience, worked with PLWHA during his time as case manager for an organization that focuses on the needs of homeless individuals. He completed an asynchronous online MSW program and was pleased with his development of clinical knowledge and skills that he uses in his current line of work, although he was not necessarily challenged in the classroom.

> Overall, I found it good. It gave me the kind of education that I was looking for, and I do think that it trained me to be able to do more clinical kinds of social work. I don't think it necessarily added anything in terms of case management or general administrative knowledge. But clinical knowledge, it did add that…It gave me access to internship spaces that I otherwise would not have been able to access…And I appreciated the flexibility of it. I did almost all of it online and I found that that did not detract at all from being able to learn or get quality education. I didn't find it a very rigorous program, which lines up with what I've read and heard that there's in general a very low barrier of entry to pursue a master's level of social work. That's not necessarily bad, it is just different doing a master's degree in analytical chemistry, for example. (Scott)

Scott's experiences contrast with that of Emma, a current MSW student who works at an organization that provides services to the PLWHA community. Emma worked full-time throughout her time in a MSW program and had her first-year practicum sponsored by her employer. While finding fault with some of her school's administrative capacities, she was overall happy with her time in school.

> I mean, I like it so far. It's a huge school and it can be unorganized. I have enjoyed the professors and the experience in class, the coursework, I think it's a thorough program. I think that we get a lot of, I mean I see [it] as a good school. You can tell when you get to see the professors and the quality of the work, but I think they could work on organization of the social work program better. But overall, I think I've enjoyed it. (Emma)

For Bryan, school was a positive and transformative experience. Their program exceeded expectations and provided them with a solid foundation upon which to develop a professional career.

> I feel very passionate about social work. Like I just think, it's why I feel going back to social work school, I was like, why doesn't everyone learn this? I was like, why isn't this the education that's in public schools? Just learning about the ways that our systems work. Like how is that not a part of regular education? So maybe that's part of the radicalization, but just how I felt so inspired by school. I don't know why, yeah, I just, I don't know why I felt a need to mention that, but just, yeah, I don't know. And school was really great. (Bryan)

While others described their programs in more tempered or ambivalent terms, Bryan's account describes a more immersive engagement with social work education. The language of "radicalization" suggests more than knowledge-building, but an orientation to values that may affect how Bryan may see their role in the profession. However, Bryan's experience diverged from that of most participants, who recognized some good instructors and classes but overall recalled their classroom education less fondly.

HIV in the Curriculum

Social work education programs fail to provide sufficient education and training about HIV. Although many programs claim to include education about the virus in coursework, commonly used textbooks and other materials often have little to no mention of HIV (Bowen, 2013; Rowan & Shears, 2011). A recent survey of social work students demonstrating low to borderline knowledge about HIV suggests students are not being taught this material (Labra et al., 2023). Almost all participants noted they received very little or outdated information about HIV in their coursework. Kate, a current MSW student completing her second-year employment-based practicum with an organization that provides a range of services to PLWHA, noted her dismay at the level of education offered by her MSW program.

> It came up once, and it came up, I remember, because I got very upset and I think I wrote to the school about how dated they were used a piece of book from 2002 and it said AIDS, didn't say HIV it just said AIDS. And it was really stigmatizing, and it was really about the danger that AIDS posed to other people. Not like the social conditions that someone living with HIV might face. Yeah, it was very terrible. (Kate)

Kate expressed concern that class materials were obsolete, incomplete, and insensitive. Kate has been employed in the HIV field for several years before pursuing her MSW. She observed a considerable gap between her passion and work with PLWHA and ineffective classroom content. Kate's experience underscores deficiencies in the preparation of social work students for work with PLWHA.

Luca, a social worker with more than five years' post-MSW experience, completed their first-year placement with an agency that served many PLWHA. They recalled little discussion about HIV in their courses, as well as inadequate education about issues pertaining to sexuality and sexual orientation.

> I think the only times we talked about it [HIV] were when I talked about my field experiences. And yeah, very poor education around queerness and essentially none around gender. Yeah, that I think is a significant area of growth for social work generally...I'm pushing for human sexuality and gender education, educational standards with CSWE...That was lacking in my program for sure and I still see it in folks I've worked with or other social workers I've interacted with. I just don't know how to talk to people about gender, about sex, about their bodies in ways that feel inviting and let a person know you don't need to feel shame about this. I want you to feel like you can talk to me about this if you so choose. (Luca)

Social work has traditionally struggled to address matters of sexuality and sexual orientation without devolving into pathology or lecturing about so-called risk behaviors (Giertsen et al., 2023; Morton et al., 2013; Newman et al., 2009). Luca's classroom experiences raise concerns that social workers will not be prepared to discuss matters of sex, gender and sexuality, limiting their effectiveness to address issues relevant to clients.

It is disappointing, but not surprising, that most participants could not recall lessons or discussion about the virus in their MSW programs.

However, some participants were introduced to HIV in their BSW programs. Paige, a current MSW student working full-time at an agency that focuses on the needs of PLWHA, recalled how an instructor brought a social policy class to life by showing a documentary about the epidemic to students.

> I had a wonderful professor that, you know, I think a lot of 21-year-olds studying social welfare, you know, social work students are not really necessarily interested in, like, the legislative parts of it. So, she was very engaging with documentaries. And the first documentary we saw in that class was *How to Survive a Plague* about the AIDS epidemic. And I have chills thinking about it now. And I rewatched it when I started my current role. And, you know, showing us the work of ACT UP New York, you know, I grew up as a queer kid in REDACTED. I really didn't know a lot about that. And also, I was born in the 90s, so HIV and AIDS were really kind of seen as over when I was growing up and not really – it really kind of connected me with the survivors of that and understanding how to serve them in my role as a social worker today. (Paige)

The documentary *How to Survive a Plague* (France, 2012) features archival footage from the earliest years of the epidemic and interviews with activists. While the film has been praised for its evocative storytelling and first-hand accounts (Holden, 2012), others have criticized its focus on White, wealthy men and the promotion of a narrative that the epidemic is finished (Schulman, 2021). For Paige, an appreciation of the history of HIV and the activism of groups such as ACT UP was an important prerequisite for her work with PLWHA; she felt more connected with her clients by gaining perspective about the early years of the epidemic. Paige also acknowledged that members of her generation (Millennials) believed that HIV was "over" and not relevant to their lives. This may speak to a lack of education and exposure to PLWHA, rather than the reality of the current state of the epidemic.

T also learned about HIV in their BSW program. They were scheduled to take a class about HIV in their MSW program, but it was cancelled due to lack of enrollment. T expressed disappointment that, despite HIV being a "huge issue" in their state, there continued to be limited discussion about the virus outside of their practicum. Despite the historical import of the HIV epidemic and its impact on social work practice, HIV was virtually ignored in the classrooms of these participants. This omission may limit opportunities for students to develop foundational knowledge about the virus and constrain their ability to situate HIV within broader socioecological contexts central to effective practice with PLWHA

Preparation for Practice

Participants were asked if their classroom learning adequately prepared them for their practicums and social work careers post-graduation. Overall, they reported that their coursework did not equip them for practice outside of academic settings. Emma, who was already working full-time with PLWHA as she pursued her MSW, believed that her in- person experiences with clients were more useful to her learning than the theories and skills introduced in the classroom.

> I think nothing prepares you more than just immersing yourself and doing it and getting that experience. I think they like, they teach a lot of CBT [Cognitive Behavioral Therapy] and MI [Motivational Interviewing] and

stuff like that. Then our beginner practice class, like Practice I and II, was more case management and social work in that case management sector focused. I feel like at that point I had already been doing the work for a few years, and so they didn't teach me anything I didn't already know. I mean, they called, they just called it different names and stuff, but I think the bulk of it I had experienced in my job. Of course I did learn some things, but I think the most of it I learned through work experience. (Emma)

Emma's account highlights once again how participants identified an uneven alignment between the realities of practice and their educational environment. From a socioecological perspective, this suggests that organizational contexts (addressed in Chapter 6) may take precedence in the education and development of early career social workers' professional identities.

Derek, a social worker with five years' post-MSW experience, was asked whether his program positioned him to for a social work career. He appreciated the community of learners he met but acknowledged that little can truly prepare early career social workers for the vicissitudes of practice.

I mean, yes and no. Yes and no, right? Like I definitely learned stuff that I utilized and applied. And I think that overall, the program did a really good job of incorporating our placements into the coursework. And also, just like community with all my students and talking about our placements and getting support. So, I felt like it went hand in hand that way that the classes, but also just sort of the community built with my cohort and what we talked about provided a lot of like support around it. But…it's very, you know, it's a lot. I don't know anything, you know, I don't know that like four years of med

> school could really prepare you. It's overwhelming. It was a place where I could come for support and help me engage with certain things, for sure. Did it adequately prepare me? I don't think it could have, you know. (Derek)

Nora, a social worker with five years' post-MSW experience, similarly described a disconnect between the clinically-focused orientation of her training and the realities she encountered in practice. She was asked whether the classroom had sufficiently prepared her for her current position in medical case management.

> I'm leaning towards no, not fully. Primarily because the program that I went to was very clinically focused. And so, a lot of my classes, at least in the second year that I remember, were very much modality focused. Let's discuss this modality, the theory behind it, the person who came up with it. And that was not the reality. In my placements and even in the work that I've done since graduating, I think it was better suited for someone who knew they were going into it to be a therapist, some sort of psychotherapy, clinical psychiatrist, or anything like that, but not for a generalist social worker I would say. (Nora)

Nora's experience suggests that students, especially those who may choose to pursue case management roles, may benefit from an advanced generalist concentration less focused on clinical mental health practice (Daley & Borasky, 2025; Dran, 2014; Lavitt, 2009).

Scott viewed the coursework component of his social work education as helpful primarily insofar as it served as an entry point into his practicum, where he felt most of his learning occurred.

> I would say yes and no. I think yes in the sense that the work that I'm doing requires a graduate degree and the internship experiences I had which really trained me I would not have had without the MSW experience. However, I would say that the actual course content of the MSW did not make much of a difference. It was things that I either already knew or had learned through homeless services work or would have learned reading on my own or through my internships. So, was it necessary? Yes, it was necessary logistically, but would I say to someone, the MSW experience, the coursework is going to be great? I would say, no, they're courses. You have to do them, but you could read the books on your own and you'll be fine. (Scott)

Scott, like Emma, derived greater value from his on-the-job social work experiences than from his time in the classroom. Overall, participants emphasized their experiences working with clients were more influential in developing their approaches to social work practice than coursework. These observations underscore the central role of experiential learning, while raising concerns that MSW programs are not meeting the needs of students.

Social Work Practicums

Practicum education has been referred to as a "signature pedagogy" of social work education (Olson-Morrison et al., 2019; Skeen, 2023; Wayne et al., 2010). The 2022 Educational Policy and Accreditation Standards (EPAS) of the Council on Social Work Education (CSWE) places a strong emphasis on the contribution of practicum learning toward the development of competent and ethical social workers.

> The [practicum] setting is where students apply human rights principles from

global and national social work ethical codes to advance social, racial, economic, and environmental justice. It fosters a learning environment where anti-racism, diversity, equity, and inclusion are valued. [Practicum] education is designed to integrate the theoretical and conceptual contributions of the explicit curriculum in the [practicum] setting. (Council on Social Work Education, 2022, p. 22)

Participants were asked to reflect upon their time in their social work practicums and share about their responsibilities, experiences with supervision, and lessons learned. This section will focus on the 11 participants who had at least one practicum placement where they had substantial interactions with PLWHA.

Practicum Responsibilities

Participants shared that they were assigned a variety of tasks during their practicums, including medical case management, psychotherapy, substance abuse screenings and support, and generalist social work tasks including providing referrals for services. Kate, who had an employment-based practicum with a large agency that specialized in providing a range of social services for PLWHA, discussed her responsibilities as a student.

> As a student intern I assist with different, so I am part of the client services team as a student intern, so in my role…in my paid job, I'm on the admin team. And so for my practicum, I'm with client services, specifically serving people living with HIV. And so I will assist with social support and client financial assistance, assisting with when someone comes in for a medical appointment, trying to get them scheduled, or confirming their insurance,

> and making sure that that is up to date in coordinating different care that they might need and trying to be a conduit for the client with the case manager that they're working with. If the case manager is not available, then I can relay messages as well as organizing food for our food bank. (Kate)

T found themself in a similar role as Kate during their second-year placement providing medical case management to PLWHA.

> When I started, I was doing more neutral tasks like providing gas vouchers for patients or writing work excuses. And as I got more, what's the word, more access to things, I was able to like update assessments, which included a bio-psycho- social [assessments] with patients. And I got to get patients connected with resources throughout the state and stuff like that. (T)

The scope of responsibilities described by Kate and T point to the inherently socioecological nature of social work with PLWHA. Their experiences demonstrate the interaction between individual client care and the broader systems that structure the availability of resources and support. Practicum settings allowed them to see how these dynamics operate in real time, a valuable learning opportunity for their professional development.

Luca recalled how busy they were in their first-year placement with an organization that offered services and resources, including harm reduction interventions, to PLWHA and individuals at risk of HIV.

> The places that I worked in primarily were with the syringe exchange and the chemical assessments...We would do these assessments to see if folks qualified to have the state subsidize, and usually they would pay for the

> entire cost, for people to attend primarily residential drug treatment. And yeah, part of it was based, or the majority of it was based on like folks' income, kind of other like aspects about their health status. So, if folks were living with HIV, they could get preference in treatment. And yeah, also taking into account some of the other like substance use factors. If folks were using, [they] were considered to be like higher risk, so using like injection equipment or injecting drugs, we could usually get them into treatment faster and usually they would qualify like almost every time for these funds because yeah, they're limited state funds. So making sure that, we wanted to try to make those available to the folks that they consider to be the most vulnerable, whether or not they actually were. That's another question. (Luca)

Luca acknowledged that for some PLWHA, their diagnosis provided them priority access to resources because they were perceived as more vulnerable and needy than their HIV-negative peers. This idea is explored in greater detail in Chapter 6.

Derek's first-year placement also involved providing harm reduction services to individuals who used substances, a substantial proportion of whom were PLWHA. He remembered the challenging nature of this work in an area of his city that had a high concentration of individuals misusing substances.

> REDACTED was a bit chaotic, which had, you know, pluses and minuses. I did a bunch of different things at first like they had a drop-in center so I was like helping out there, literally like they had bathrooms in the drop-in center so I'd have to monitor the bathrooms, you know, keep time, make sure people weren't in there too long…like make sure they weren't like

> overdosing you know. I did that. And eventually, gratefully, they started the first mobile suboxone program in REDACTED. And I was sort of the assistant. They had a care manager, they had a doctor, they had a driver, and I was just sort of the assistant. So that's what I did. (Derek)

During Derek's second-year practicum, he was placed with a community mental health center that had a specialized program for PLWHA. At this organization, he was able to gain experience developing clinical skills.

> So, one half I was you know, I'm a therapist and had a few patients on outpatient weekly basis, and the other half support staff for REDACTED. And my big thing was I hosted a weekly group that I could do anything with. And I just, I called it like Poz Topics, like Hot Topics, but like different relevant topics around HIV and AIDS and we would just, you know, provide some education around it, whatever it was, and yeah, sort of host the group processing. (Derek)

While both of Derek's practicums involved working with PLWHA, the settings and nature of the work differed considerably. Social work with PLWHA extends beyond medical issues to include a range of psychosocial supports situated within multiple community contexts, reflecting the nature of the epidemic in the post-ART era. This diversity of practice expands the scope of skills required of social workers engaged with PLWHA.

Bryan's first-year placement was as a housing case manager at a large organization that provided a host of services to PLWHA. They did not find this work to be particularly meaningful.

> I was a case manager and so I essentially worked with people who were given an apartment and who had been previously homeless. And having a serious mental illness and being diagnosed with HIV/AIDS was also one of the requirements to getting an apartment…We had to do weekly check-ins, which really were just like, how are you doing? Like, it really wasn't much. And to be honest, so much of that job is about collecting paperwork, sadly. I think that is sort of the nature of a lot of non-profits. So much of it is just about proving that you're doing the work. And so, it's trying to collect lab results from people, making sure that they're staying within all the eligibility requirements to maintain their housing. So much of it is about upkeep rather than direct care. (Bryan)

During their second-year placement, Bryan transitioned to another organization that offers services to LGBTQ+ communities. They was assigned to the behavioral health department and provided psychotherapy to a wide range of clients, including approximately 6 PLWHA.

> I was fully a psychotherapist. And so, and they really gave us free rein to use whatever kind of treatment modalities we wanted to, interventions, like really utilizing, you know, trying to get to know our own styles from the things we've learned in school and stuff. And there still being a nonprofit, lots of assessments, like lots of a very long, like a very lengthy intake process in terms of assessments and questions and also a lot of like upkeep of every three months having to reassess people for different things. But otherwise, the role was really just like a therapist of just weekly seeing people for 45 minutes and doing my notes. (Bryan)

The practicum responsibilities described by Bryan and other participants reflect experiences typical of social work practicums. However, work with PLWHA introduced a wide range of socioecological factors that distinguished these experiences from more generalist practice contexts.

Practicum Supervision

Supervision of students' practicum experience is an essential element of their learning (Bogo, 2014; Ketner et al., 2017; Zuchowski et al., 2021). The CSWE EPAS (2022) states that MSW programs must ensure that students receive supervision in their practicums from an individual who holds a master's degree in social work and has at least two years of post-master's degree social work practice experience. The supervisory relationship reflects the life course principle of linked lives, as the guidance of experienced practitioners influences how early career social workers understand their roles and future trajectories in the profession (Carr, 2018). Participants described considerable variation in structure and quality of practicum supervision. Luca, whose first practicum was spent working with individuals with substance use concerns, remembered consulting their supervisor for guidance on how to respond to clients' questions about their own using history. Their supervisor offered good suggestions and gave them the freedom to decide what was appropriate when it came to disclosure. Luca also recalled a time when they witnessed a client who had overdosed. Their supervisor, who was not present during the incident, made sure to call Luca, checked in on their welfare, and offered them a day off if necessary. Luca was appreciative of this support, noting "that was a really helpful example…of the kind of care that we should expect and can offer each other…doing this kind of work" (Luca). Luca remarked that their supervisor saw them as a person first, a social worker second. This type of care and concern reflects a relational approach to supervision in which learning and professional development take precedence over task compliance.

T shared how their supervisor helped them tackle overwhelming tasks.

> I get lost very easily, and the way that the clinic is set up, it is a maze, it feels like. And so, I would easily be able to find a social worker and be like, hey, I have no idea where I'm going, could you help me? And with my supervisor, she was incredibly supportive and really pushed me to be the best version of myself and the best social worker I could be. I have a lot of areas where I know that I struggle with, like phone calls. I really suck at phone calls. I have hearing issues. And so, like for me, I have to really listen and really focus in order to do phone calls. And she would like frequently push me to be making phone calls and to help her with her voicemails and call back on clients and respond to them without her assistance. Because even though I felt like I didn't know the answers, I did know the answers, and I could provide support and assistance for these patients. (T)

Supervision offered T a chance to work on specific tasks and gain confidence and emotional support from a trusted individual at a developmentally sensitive time in their educational and career trajectories. T felt "the best version of myself and the best social worker I could be", highlighting the power of effective supervision for students who may doubt their abilities.

Vanessa worked with PLWHA in both her BSW and MSW practicums where her supervisors had contrasting approaches to supervision. Experiencing both styles helped her identify what kinds of supervisory supports were most useful to her as she developed her practice.

> I shared an office with my [BSW practicum] supervisor. She was very sweet, very accessible. She held an LMSW credential. She was more of a behind the scenes supervisor. She told me my assignment, but she wasn't really as like, okay, give me an example of how you would talk to a patient. She wasn't hands-on, but she was still good overall. And then for my current placement, she was kind of opposite. She was a lot more hands-on, a lot more like, okay, how did you feel about this? How would you do something differently? And just more trying to make me think more and be able to apply that in a practical setting. (Vanessa)

The experiences of Luca, T, and Vanessa speak to the two of the three essential functions of practicum supervision—educational instruction and emotional support (the third being administrative oversight) (Hylton & Manit, 2020). Effective supervision benefits both supervisors and students. When supervisors draw upon their past and present professional experiences, their feedback, informed by their practice wisdom, enhances students' learning. Providing supervision also gives supervisors opportunities to develop leadership and management skills that inform their future career paths (Ketner et al., 2017).

However, other participants related that their supervisors were overworked and overwhelmed with their own responsibilities and did not have adequate time to provide consistent, meaningful supervision.

> I would say it would focus on more client questions I had. So, I would come with a list of so-and-so says they need this, do you know of a referral? And then otherwise, there wasn't a lot of support. I think, like my supervisor was

> really overworked and just didn't have a lot of capacity to answer specific questions. (Issa)

Derek also found his supervisor to be unavailable, so he leaned into other staff members to provide him with guidance and support.

> Unfortunately, my supervisor had a very casual approach to supervision, and he was great, but we wouldn't meet regularly. Yeah, I think if I was younger, or maybe didn't have the lived experience I have, I might have been overwhelmed or something. But luckily, you know, there's just a lot of great people on staff there that I turn to for support when needed, but I didn't get really great supervision there. (Derek)

Derek drew upon a reservoir of personal experience to compensate for the lack of supervision; however, this does not conform with CSWE requirements regarding the signature pedagogy of practicum education. The absence of consistent and structured supervision limits opportunities to integrate and process interactions with clients and possibly impedes professional development. Bryan was unimpressed with their supervisor from their first-year placement and recalled a particularly unpleasant encounter.

> I did not love my supervisor at REDACTED…she was not a social worker. Like, I don't even know what her degrees were. It was more like she was like an administrator, just like trying to keep the housing department running. And often I don't think that she had clinical wisdom. Like one time, one of my clients literally came in and like, this is a man who's homeless, she literally told him he looked dirty and that next time he came to the office, he should

> like try and look better. And like, it definitely was in that moment where I was like, yeah, I don't trust anything you say. (Bryan)

Overall, the uneven, varied experiences of supervision reported by participants suggests that the signature pedagogy of social work is not receiving the attention it warrants and calls into question the profession's ability to prepare early career social workers for the demands of practice.

Lessons Learned

Most participants enjoyed their practicums working with PLWHA and shared they gained in-depth knowledge about the functions of social work and the operations of medical and social services organizations. Ashley, a social worker with more than five years' post-MSW experience, had both her BSW and MSW practicums with organizations that provided services to PLWHA. She gained a new appreciation for the difficulties PLWHA experience when dealing with health care organizations.

> Probably my favorite thing was being able to witness the way that the medical field operates and how it's just inherently incompatible with like the social needs of people...Like for example, the medical system...was kind of designed for a patient who's, you know, quote unquote compliant, White, thin, has money, like can understand like the jargon. I've learned that the people, the providers, the specialists would either talk to the clients like they were stupid or they would use language that I would even have to look up or they would talk to me instead of the client if I was in the room... I'm driving them home and I'm like, how was that for you? Do those instructions make sense? Like can you do that? Because they'll be like, oh, eat this, or do that, or put this medication in the fridge. I was like, this person's fridge hasn't been working

> for three weeks. Like the practical kind of follow-through was really interesting for me to coordinate. Yeah, so that's what I liked about it. (Ashley)

In describing the failings of medical systems, Ashley recognized that the health of her clients was not just a matter for doctors. Her practicum learning offered her familiarity with the broader socioecological factors that allowed her to situate client care within broad frameworks, an approach she continues to employ in her medical case management work with PLWHA.

Issa learned they did not enjoy case management. However, they appreciated learning about an innovative housing model at their practicum where PLWHA lived together in an apartment complex that also housed the social work department.

> I would say a lot about how nonprofits function and how federal funding interacts with a nonprofit's programs, dictating what they can offer. I loved the housing model of having community in that space and that was something that I actually still think about, like I would love to work in another setting within social work where people are living together. That was meaningful to me. I sort of confirmed that case management was challenging for me and not as meaningful. But I really admire, there were some people who had been doing case management for several years, and their clients loved them. And I could tell, like, they were just so kind and generous. So, a lot of respect for the people. (Issa)

T shared that their practicum experience helped them to develop important social work skills in engaging with both clients and medical providers and gain confidence in their professional development.

On a professional level, it really helped me to develop the skills of empathy and continuous care, but also knowing where to stop. I love the patients that I got to interact with throughout my year there. And I am incredibly sad that I am no longer gonna be there next semester and I hope to get a job there…And I think it really taught me just how to work with other people which is a skill that I'm not that great at…I tend to just say things or I tend to be an independent worker and the collaboration that I was able to do at the clinic was amazing. Like I was able to approach the providers and be like, hey, you can't do that with this patient.

They won't want to do it. (T)

Participants were generally satisfied with their experiences in placements working with PLWHA. The practicum learning comprised two distinct but related areas. First, participants learned about the individual-level skills and knowledge standard of good social work practice. And second, they appreciated how social work systems and organizations operate in real time.

Necessary Knowledge and Skills

Participants were asked what skills and knowledge were necessary for social workers engaged with PLWHA. Consistently, participants shared that social workers should have an understanding of the history of the HIV epidemic and the psychosocial issues encountered by clients. There was less discussion about the medical aspects of the virus. Historical awareness enables social workers to situate clients' experiences with HIV within the broader arc of pivotal moments and shifting social conditions that affect how their lives unfold. Issa believed social workers should seek out resources about the history of the epidemic.

> I think definitely some of the cultural information, especially anything you can get from people who actually experience the HIV/AIDS epidemic, and just understanding like how widespread it was, how scary it was, how non-responded to by the government it was. Oh, something I learned that really bothered me was how Ryan White is the name of this federal funding for HIV support and basically the poster child for it was this young white teenager who, I hope I'm getting this right, got HIV through blood transfusion, I think, rather than actually sort of like, actually the predominant experience of that time, which was queer people, like gay men and trans women, who were really marginalized in so many ways. So instead, it was like sort of this very privileged and unusual face of like, providing support to HIV positive people. That was something I learned, and I would want other people to know. But yeah, I mean there's so many like books and movies, documentaries about that time and then the like basic medical information about medications, what it means to be undetectable and the, you know, like safety and freedom you have being undetectable and things like, you know, all the ways that you can't get HIV that people are worried about, crap, yeah, things like that. (Issa)

While Issa mentioned the appreciation of "basic medical information", their response focused more on how PLWHA were marginalized and failed by governments and health systems. They also mentioned Ryan White, the namesake of the groundbreaking legislation that continues to provide substantial support to PLWHA and the organizations that serve them. The media's portrayal of White, a young White male who became infected with HIV through a blood transfusion, as an avatar of the epidemic obscured the identities of those who were most impacted by HIV—sexual minority men and people of color (Esparza, 2019; Renfro, 2024). Given that most social workers working with PLWHA will undoubtedly have some involvement with the Ryan White CARE Act, Issa felt strongly about the importance of this history.

Bryan was conflicted whether social workers needed to understand the medical aspects of HIV. They believed that social workers should possess some knowledge about viral loads and CD4 counts, but recognized that social workers are not typically expected to comprehend the medical specifics of other chronic conditions.

> I mean, a basic understanding of CD4 counts and what numbers constitute what may be a problem. I think having a basic understanding of our immune system and what the disease is is helpful. I think having a knowledge of medications too and how effective they are, I think that's really important because obviously there's just a lot of fear around having it. So, it's like to have the knowledge of treatments, I think is really important for people to have their anxieties and fears soothed. I don't know, but to be honest, I don't know if I feel it is that important to have because even so, I feel there's still a lot I don't necessarily understand about how it all works biologically speaking but that's not to say I feel I couldn't help people deal with it and I guess I'm thinking about I have clients who have cancer and it's not like I really have a working understanding of cancer and cancer treatments but I do feel I'm helping them yeah so I don't know about that one. I guess like,

> yes and no in a way, that you have to have that info. (Bryan)

Bryan believed that they could provide services to their PLWHA clients without grasping the underlying science. There is an important distinction between biomedical expertise and social work support, but a basic understanding of the virus may assist social workers contextualize treatment, explain the importance of adherence, and effectively advocate for clients.

Other participants stated that social workers working with PLWHA must engage in reflexive practice and uphold the values and ethical standards of the profession. When asked about the knowledge and skills necessary for practice with PLWHA, Vanessa mentioned "empathy, cultural sensitivity, how to communicate on all levels, on all educational levels, being respectful, not having any bias and being able to advocate for them". Along these same lines, Kate believed that social workers must assume an anti- oppressive approach to social work practice.

> To me, it is really critical self-reflection and considering your own biases, and I think that the way that it comes up in like my job, a lot is like a client might seem difficult in some way. And if we're practicing anti-oppressive social work, then we need to ask ourselves why we would be considering that client difficult in what systems of oppression, such as homophobia or racism, transphobia, like anything that might be really making us view this person in a way that is changing our perspective of them and also what that means to be difficult could that also just be self-advocacy…It's not like we can't blame an individual for their circumstance if we want to be, I mean to me a successful and compassionate social worker isn't going to look at a person and say, you have failed all these ways, shame on you. Don't be a social worker if you feel

that way. (Kate)

For Kate, a necessary skill for social workers, particularly those working with PLWHA, is recognizing that clients' resistance or noncompliance must be understood within the totality of their past experiences and the intersecting systems of oppression shaping their lives. This perspective reframes client behaviors as responses to socioecological limitations. This knowledge can serve as an important foundation for the professional development of early career social workers by enhancing their capacity for responsive practice.

Self-Care

Self-care, broadly construed as activities designed to alleviate personal and professional stressors, is an ethical obligation for social workers. The NASW Code of Ethics (2021) states "professional self-care is paramount for competent and ethical social work practice. Professional demands, challenging workplace climates, and exposure to trauma warrant that social workers maintain personal and professional health, safety, and integrity" (p. 4). Social work scholars and practitioners have explored the conceptualization of self-care and incorporation of these activities into the lives of social workers (Lee & Miller, 2013; Ratcliff, 2024; Shepherd & Newell, 2020). Bressi and Vaden (2017) offer the following definition of self-care.

> Self-care is inclusive of agentic self-regulated activities that purposefully a.) bolster the ability to sit within, tolerate and understand the affective and identity dysregulation related to experiencing vulnerability and uncertainty in the social work relationship, and b.) make meaning of the ways workers' selves are changed from work with clients. (p. 37)

They argue that some approaches to self-care are based on the view of the self as divided into professional and personal domains, with equilibrium maintained through protective boundaries between the two. While acknowledging some benefits to this method of self-care, Bressi and Vaden (2017) warn social workers may be discouraged from any use of the self in their work with clients. Participants were asked to share their self-care strategies and practices in their work with PLWHA. They noted the importance of creating both physical and mental distance from their work as a major element of their self-care. Nora strove not to take her work home with her, but found this to be difficult in practice.

> Yeah, I try not to take my work home with me. I don't have Teams or our remote phone system on my cell phone. I really try to keep those very separate. If I'm not here I don't want to know. That's how I feel. Which is hard because we're working with people, you know, this is not like data. These are not Excel spreadsheets. And so, part of it is there's guilt there as well. So yeah, it's hard. I don't know. I don't know what...there's always talk about self-care in our work and yeah, I'm conflicted about that language and, you know, the feeling of ownership over that when it's a systemic issue. Like if the systems existed and I could get my clients support, maybe I wouldn't feel this way. And some of those feelings are just hard to mitigate with a bath, you know. (Nora)

Nora noted that the rhetoric of self-care often encourages individual-level interventions that fail to address the root cause of stress—the frustrations of not being able to meet the needs of clients. When Nora stated that her clients are not "data" or

“Excel spreadsheets”, she implied that her that her clients are not abstract concepts, but real people with real problems. Nora believed that her work has meaning and value, which only compounded her stress.

Winnie, a recent MSW graduate with less than two years’ experience, also highlighted the importance of maintaining guardrails between their job and home life.

> I definitely try to be very intentional about self-care. One thing that I really appreciate about REDACTED, in this position I guess specifically, is that it is a very, very strict 9-5 job…I can know like I will come home, I will, you know, be home at 5pm, and I do not have to think about work anymore. And I have been relatively good about that. (Winnie)

Winnie observed that their self-care is facilitated by organizational policies, such as a strict 9:00am-5:00pm daily schedule. This suggests that self-care is not just a matter of individual responsibility, but also an organizational priority meant to promote wellbeing and career sustainability.

Like Winnie, Ashley stressed her need for boundaries between her personal and professional lives.

> Boundaries. I have always been really good about boundaries, specifically in terms of nine to five kind of stuff. Like after five o'clock, I'm not looking at, sometimes I do if I have to, if I'm at work, it's been a crazy day, but what I'll do is I'll work less the next day. So, time boundaries are super important to me. Like work is work, home is home. (Ashley)

Ashley’s comment that “work is work, home is home” demonstrates how she perceives self-care as an effort to maintain homeostasis between two selves—the professional ("work") and personal ("home").

Many participants indicated that psychotherapy was their preferred self-care activity. Paige shared that psychotherapy, in conjunction with medication, played a major role in her self-care.

> I will start by saying most, if not every social worker, has a reason they got into the field, right? So, I certainly have a background rooted in trauma, and therapy is a must attend for me. I have been in weekly therapy on and off for 15 years, and that's, you know, especially in the kind of work I do, I think it's very important. So that's number one. I also take SSRIs, which is new to me. I was not on any medication within the last three months, actually, in therapy I realized that it's because, like many other social workers, I was kind of throwing myself into other people's problems for a long time. But now I'm in a role that's manageable and I'm not overwhelmed all the time. And so, my kind of anxiety caught up with me this year because I was able to manage it better. So being proactive about that has been really helpful. (Paige)

Paige recognized that the challenges of her role, in conjunction with past trauma, makes therapy essential to her self-care. Other participants found support and comfort in community with colleagues and friends. Ashley used her consultation group as a way to vent about work in ways that she could not do because of supervisory responsibilities.

> I'm in a supervision group for clinical licensure and it's all medical social workers. Half of us are with REDACTED. So just being like, you guys, this is crazy. And then being like, yeah, that's crazy is really helpful for me to kind of commiserate because one of the things that I noticed, this is my first

supervisory role. When you're a supervisor, you can't talk crap about people to your staff. Like you can't say my staff person, Staff A sucks. I can't engage in that kind of workplace stuff…I think those are the big ones, being able to share my experiences and commiserate with, not commiserate, that sounds bad, but like relate to other people and kind of offload a little bit and maintaining those boundaries for sure. (Ashley)

Ashley could rely upon close counsel with trusted colleagues when she cannot be frank with her supervisees. In her current role, she does not receive much supervision; her professional network gives her the space to process work-related matters and maintain healthy boundaries.

Tony, a social worker with five years' post-MSW experience, touched upon all three of the previous strategies (work/life balance; psychotherapy; support from friends) to describe their approach to self-care.

I think really focusing on what are the things within and outside of my control. And yeah, not overextending myself in terms of staying late or having some good boundaries around that. And then, you know, I see my own therapist, and I think I, it's helpful. Like a lot of my friends are in social work. And so, we understand what our today is like. And yeah, and I don't, I try not to talk or vent about work at home just because I think it kind of, it doesn't always feel productive. (Tony)

Participants recalled how challenging self-care could be when trying to juggle the demands of school, practicum, and outside employment. Emma expressed gratitude that her MSW journey was coming to a close and acknowledged the stress of balancing school, work, and personal lives.

> It's been hard. I think it's not, like, it's not sustainable. So I'm glad it's almost over. I think for the most part, I try to take opportunities to rest when I can and exercise when I can and allow myself to no matter how much I have to do, reserve time for myself and like my social life once a week. It's definitely tough, though. I think just like kind of getting ahead of it before I feel I'm burnt out, too. Like when I kind of notice it coming on, scheduling a day off, a day of rest, whatever I need, before it gets to that point of burnout has been helpful. (Emma)

Emma used the term "burnout". Defined as a state of prolonged stress characterized by exhaustion, cynicism, and lowered professional effectiveness, burnout is not uncommon for social work students (Benner & Curl, 2018; Powell & Mayfield, 2024;

Robins et al., 2018). When asked what might have helped her address potential burnout, Emma shared that she was not able to take advantage of her program's support services because she was not on campus until evenings. She believed more flexible classroom policies would be of greatest benefit.

> I think it depends with attendance and stuff policies. They, I think that they could be a little bit better about giving us maybe one mental health class per semester, especially for the part-time program, given that a lot of us do work, and that's why we're there. Like I work all day and then I go to class until 8:20 and I don't even have time to like eat sometimes. So I think there's, I think, yeah, I think they could be a little bit more gracious with that. That

would be nice. (Emma)

Bryan, a recent graduate, remembered how challenging it was to engage in the types of self-care activities they enjoyed due to financial constraints and the conflicting messages they received from their program about self-care.

> School was a lot…In terms of self-care throughout all of that, I feel like I could have done a better job. I'm very into like fitness and working out…it definitely really decreased throughout school, but I definitely tried to work out a lot and exercise. One of the jobs I had was at a gym. I was in the front desk, so I got to take free classes there. So that definitely helped. But then by the end of the last semester, I was too overwhelmed. I had to quit because I had so much to do and I wanted to give everything to school...Yeah, I think right now, and actually this is sort of emblematic throughout school, like I just need money. Like if I had money, I could like buy the fitness classes I want to go take. I could go get a massage. Like I think a lot of the things that I do in my self-care are expensive, which like, I know I could change that view and do other things, but yeah, I think it just was really hard because you're so ill-resourced during school, typically, as I was, and it's not easy to take care of ourselves. And they tell you to, but it's like, you guys are giving us so much work. (Bryan)

Bryan recognized that their self-care was constrained not just by personal preferences, but also by a lack of adequate funds and an academic/work schedule that did not allow them sufficient time. Self-care is not simply an individual responsibility, but rather a practice that is also shaped by the organizational and policy contexts that structure social work practice.

Impact of the Work on the Social Worker

Participants discussed how their experiences working with PLWHA impacted them both professionally and personally. Most participants found their work with PLWHA meaningful and rewarding. Viewed through a life course lens, these experiences represent early career turning points that contribute to the ongoing formation of professional identity and commitment to particular areas of practice (Elder Jr et al., 2003). Ashley has been interested in working with PLWHA since she was in high school and her entire career post-MSW has involved this population.

> So, what I like to tell people is that REDACTED really shaped who I am as a social worker. Like I had an interest in the LGBT community…I've always had an interest in that population, but then when I got into REDACTED, I was 22. I didn't know what was happening at all. I was told from the beginning, if you can do this job, you can do anything. And I really just fell into this medical role and being able to, I think how it's changed me is like being able to recognize the way that the system is built versus how people receive care. (Ashley)

Ashley's reflection captures how early exposure to practice settings can solidify skill development, professional competence, and awareness of socioecological factors. For T, their work with PLWHA affirmed their choice of social work as a vocation.

> And on a personal level, it really reminded me on why I chose the field of social work. It solidified for me, like, this is the field I'm meant to be in,

working with these people, even on the bad days where I – like one week at the clinic, literally every day that I was there, someone told me about their suicide attempt, which is a lot for one week, that's not normal. And I was like feeling like super bad about it because the emotional weight of that is a lot. But like despite those weeks, like I was just reminded like, this is why I'm meant to be here. Like these are the people that I'm, like, these are the types of people that I want to continue to work with. I want to be able to care for these people. And it's just like a reminder, even on the bad days, like, there's still so much good that you're able to do. (T)

Even when faced with tough situations, T made meaning of their interactions with clients and asserted their developing social worker identity. T enjoyed their practicum so much that they hoped to continue with their organization post-graduation, potentially influencing their emerging professional trajectory. Their enthusiasm suggests that positive practicum experiences can lead to future career intentions, positioning practicum settings as important sites for professional development.

Some participants shared how important it was to work in predominantly queer spaces. For Luca, their time in practicum was an opportunity to explore how they could be an authentically queer social worker.

I love to continue to work with those folks and working with queer and trans people. That has continued and that just built even more over time and that's yeah, folks I really love to work with and I think part of it started there. I don't currently work within a very queer environment. It's still a great place, but I realized how it does feel very different to be around, like, working with

> and around other queer people. And that is definitely something I want more of in my life and in my future and realized that that was something that I could have too and that I could grow even more within that. And my queerness and my identity as a queer person and my identity as a social worker don't have to be separate identities. They can exist together and that can actually be beneficial too and not just a thing that like, try to have be in there, but like, is like, either neutral or a hindrance. (Luca)

Despite the profession's orientation toward social justice, social workers find that educational and practice environments are not always queer-friendly (Arguello, 2019; Atteberry-Ash et al., 2019). Luca's positive experiences sharing their queerness with others was a life event that played an important role in their developing approach to social work practice. As discussed in the next chapter, Luca and other participants also learned about uses of self-disclosure during their time working with PLWHA.

Participants revealed that working with PLWHA made them more empathetic and accepting of others.

> It made me see things differently, especially for homeless people because I was I would be able to learn more of their everyday struggles and just…it's given me like a softer heart, more compassionate towards homeless people. I've already been passionate to them but even more…And it just irritates me when I see stuff online of like stigma around or stereotypes around HIV. I just feel more educated about it, more passionate about it. So, I'd say I feel stronger in my beliefs. (Vanessa)

However, some participants stated that their time working with PLWHA had opened their eyes to systemic issues that negatively affect their clients. Tony expressed concern that even with their best efforts, their clients may still not be able to meet their needs.

> I think it really plays into kind of the moral injury that comes up with like doing this work and that you are often with folks who have been deeply disenfranchised and then the resources don't exist that would dramatically change their situation. Like, I think I do offer everything I know and even if it's not my role, if they want to talk about housing, we can talk about housing. I refer them to every place I know. But I think it's often like a harm reduction situation of supporting people and figuring out the least worst option. And that can take a mental toll and likely lead to burn out. (Tony)

> When asked how they define moral injury, Tony provided the following response. I think it's functioning in a system that perpetuates harm and participating in that harm. And I think there's, yeah, there's an element of, you do the best you can with the resources you have, but with the knowledge that it's like far from enough. And that there's always going to be, yeah, a power dynamic within that as well. (Tony)

Tony's use of moral injury is compatible with the concept of moral distress, the ethical dilemmas helping professionals encounter when restrictive practice environments prevent them from assisting their clients in the manner they prefer (Lynch & Forde, 2016; Weinberg, 2009). In a similar vein, Issa's practicum experience taught them the perils of burnout.

> I think it made me concerned about burnout in a social work career. There's definitely something I learned about setting boundaries with the work that I was going to do and sort of like concern I had for coworkers. Yeah. I wish that I felt I learned more. I think it was okay overall but probably more in-person interaction with clients and more supervision would probably have helped me learn more. (Issa)

For all participants, even those who had uneven or negative experiences in their organizations, there was gratitude for the opportunity to work with PLWHA and great respect and admiration for the resilience demonstrated by their clients. While each participant had a unique set of circumstances that brought them to the social work profession, they found their time working with PLWHA to be rewarding and aligned with their personal and professional values and ethics, as well as a significant milestone in their career trajectories.

Conclusion

An examination of individual-level factors within the socioecological model stresses the essential role of the self in forming social work practice with PLWHA. The thoughts, emotions, values, and experiences that social workers bring to their roles affect how they interpret client needs and sustain empathy in challenging situations. Centering individual-level factors serves as a reminder that effective social work practice begins with a thorough understanding of the person behind the professional role.

Chapter 5

Interpersonal-Level Engagement with PLWHA

The interpersonal factors of the socioecological model serve as a bridge from the personal attributes and values of the social worker to the broader organizational, community, and sociopolitical contexts that frame social work practice. In the SEM proposed for this study, the interpersonal factors focus on the vibrant and complex relationships that develop between the social worker and their clients. The participants in this study worked with PLWHA of all ages, races, sexual orientations, gender identities, disability statuses, and many other identities and experience. The work with PLWHA occurred across many settings and the goals of the work were as varied as the client demographics. Because both social workers and their clients are situated within particular historical moments and life stages, attention to life course perspectives also informs how generational position and timing impacts interpersonal dynamics. Seven themes frame this chapter: maintenance of clients' HIV care; challenges and barriers experienced by clients; client strengths and resources; the nature and use of the helping relationship; generational differences between client cohorts; the salience of HIV in the lives of clients; and social workers' uses of self-disclosure with their clients.

Client HIV Care

For participants, especially those in medical case management positions, their clients' HIV care was a significant issue, but often not the most important. Participants reported that most of their clients' viral loads were suppressed and CD4 counts were in the normal range, indicating good maintenance of their HIV. When asked about her clients' HIV care, Paige shared that on her caseload, most clients are doing well.

> In general, yes…A lot of my clients were diagnosed in the 1990s, right? So when they were diagnosed, they thought their life was over and today they're in their 60s or 70s and, you know, they take one pill a day. So they're like all over it. There are, you know, there's some, just because somebody's viral load is high doesn't necessarily mean that they're not adherent. You know, we have some, I have some folks with like sero-resistance or, you know, whatever. Some of that does come from having, you know, going on and off your meds. But for the most part, I would say definitely most of my folks are really, I would say probably 80% are really adherent and well-managed and remain undetectable on their own. I have no issues about it or like concerns with them. (Paige)

Older PLWHA have generally good knowledge about the risks of medication non-compliance, which is rooted in their own past non-compliance and knowledge accumulated over the worst years of the epidemic (Pack et al., 2023). By observing that her older clients are "like all over it", Paige implied her clients have developed a strong commitment to adherence to the point where medications have become routine.

Lynn, a social worker with more than two years' post-MSW experience but who has only been working with PLWHA for less than six months, noted their clients' HIV health was generally good with some exceptions.

> I'd say most of my clients, their numbers are well managed and they're like suppressed as far as their viral load, CD4 is good, you know, in the healthy counts and everything. I'd say the only clients where that there's…something's a little off,

> their CD4 is a little low, are people who are in recovery sometimes too, because, you know, maybe they fall back for whatever reason and like that affects, you know, I think people who just have a lot of stress going on, I noticed that as well, and we talk about that, as far as homelessness. (Lynn)

Lynn's observation suggests her understanding that health outcomes are closely connected to broader socioecological conditions and social determinants of health. Clinical indicators such as CD4 counts serve as markers of HIV health and as well as evidence of the instability and hardships experienced by clients.

Participants acknowledged the limits of their role regarding their clients' overall health, especially as it relates to HIV care. Jenny, a recent graduate with less than two years' post-MSW experience, said it was important for her to remember her clients have the right to make their own decisions regarding their health.

> You know, as a social worker, I feel like I can only do so much to try to encourage my clients to take their medications or to do certain things. But once they leave my office and go home, I can't necessarily dictate what they are doing with or how they are taking their medications. So it's kind of hard to think about how I can continue to help them when I've, you know, exhausted all my resources. (Jenny)

Jenny spoke to the frustrations many social workers experience when they feel they have done all they can for a client, yet the client does not make use of the support offered. The NASW Code of Ethics (2021) states that social workers should respect and promote the right of clients to self-determination. Jenny acknowledged this ethical mandate, even if inaction and inattention to their health may result in bad outcomes for clients. Her awareness of the boundaries of the social worker role reflects professional development and her integration of social work values.

Paige shared a similar experience as Jenny. She contextualized her predicament with a client, situating it within the history of the epidemic and the values of the social work profession.

> You know, I have a client who has never ever taken meds and won't. And, you know…this client has a declining T cell count. And we have tried to explain, you know, you, especially when you're sleeping rough, right? Like you could catch a cold and die and…you're only in your 50s or whatever. Like we can impress upon them the consequences, but, you know, we're never ever going to force, especially the population we're working with. You know, many of them have history of incarceration. Many of them, you know, are survivors of the AIDS epidemic where, you know, they were brutalized for being gay, they were brutalized for being sick, they watched all their friends die, you know, things like that. Or they're, you know, there's – I can't make anybody do anything… I try to approach my role as a collaborator. And, you know, I really try to de-center myself as an authority figure and try to take a role of somebody that truly cares about you and just wants to make sure that you're good. (Paige)

While Paige was concerned about her client's health, she recognized that coercive measures would be unethical and counterproductive. Her perspective demonstrates an awareness of the history of the epidemic and acknowledges that clients' past traumas and experiences of oppression may negatively influence how they perceive offers of assistance. It is more important for Paige to maintain a collaborative helping relationship with her client than cause a rupture over medications. For many participants, clients' adherence to HIV medications was one of the most important yet challenging aspects of their jobs.

Medication Adherence

Participants reported that supporting their clients' adherence to medication regimes was a central component of their work. Leo, a social worker with less than two years' post-MSW experience, stated that in their work as a medical case manager, the "main goal is treatment adherence". Winnie, a supervisor of medical case managers with a small caseload of their own, noted that the collection of adherence data was mandated as part of their organization's funding.

> Yes, and that's definitely kind of the main goal of medical case management, to have clients be treatment adherent and engaging in their HIV medical care. The majority of clients are on medication and are treatment adherent. Case managers are required to do quarterly treatment adherence checks with their clients. You can do that in a variety of ways, just to check in on whether clients are engaging in their medical care. (Winnie)

August recalled his time working with young people living with HIV. Constant questions about medication adherence felt intrusive and uncomfortable. He worried how this might adversely impact his relationship with clients.

> Yeah, so I would say I thought a lot about stigma in my work specifically with youth around their medication and just like, because that was a huge part of my role was, how do I get my patients to take their meds? Like, it's so annoying that that was like, it felt like my job was the med police...Yeah, I hated that part because I felt every time I asked about it, they're like, this is all he really freaking

> cares about? He only cares if I'm taking my meds or not? But that was something I had to make sure I documented every single time. So I feel I had to find creative ways to insert that somewhere in my check-ins with clients, either on the phone or in person when they were there for an appointment. (August)

August's use of "med police" is particularly interesting. The term implies aggressive surveillance and a punitive approach fundamentally at odds with social work values. August connected organizational and policy factors to adherence, illustrating a socioecological perspective. One way he was able to resolve this tension was the use of inventive methods of data collection. There are substantial historical intersections between HIV and the criminal justice system, and many PLWHA have been targets of arrest and prosecution due to their marginalized identities and serostatus (Hoppe, 2023; Quinn et al., 2024; Sanders et al., 2012). The monitoring of the medication adherence of PLWHA may be experienced in very different ways from what social workers intend.

Participants shared the constant struggle with some clients over medication adherence was one of the most frustrating parts of their jobs. Emma noted that in her experience, adherence was associated with greater challenges.

> It can be tough because it's a lot of times some of the solutions, maybe they have tried and it's really kind of bigger than that. Usually I feel like with medication adherence issues, you know, there's other things happening and it might be tied to substance use or other mental health issues, or if you're like unhoused, you know, you're getting your medication stolen. So, those are things that are hard to have conversations about. So it's tough. It's probably like the hardest part of the job. I think it also just is, at that point, also, I think it becomes a conversation of like,

what are some other things that we can work on? And what are some other services that I can offer you that might promote that adherence at the end of the day? Because, clearly, the reminders and the alarms are not working, especially when you don't have a phone. So that's just kind of how I approach it. (Emma)

Emma recognized she is constrained by a lack of effective interventions that she can offer clients around their medication use, especially when those clients are without necessary resources, such a telephone or stable housing.

T expressed what appeared to be contradictory approaches with clients who did not adhere to medication schedules. While T believed that their clients did not fully grasp the importance of taking their pills regularly, they also asserted that non-adherence was a conscious choice of their clients.

> There are many clients who just don't understand the severity of not taking their medication every day or taking the medication some days but not every day, like every other day, like it prevents it from working. And so many patients just don't understand the risks that they have in doing that. And it's understanding that they are choosing this way. And there are so many patients of mine who are going through active addiction or they want to ignore their status, so they don't want to come to the doctor. And it's knowing that, like, you're trying your best to help them get in care and continue in care and get the help that they need and help them understand what's going on with their HIV status, but it's knowing that they're choosing what they're choosing, and you can only do so much with them. (T)

For T, arriving at the realization that clients possess self-determination and remain in charge of the helping process was a significant milestone in their professional development.

Paige believed that there are generational differences among her clients when it comes to medication adherence. She recognized that her younger clients did not come of age during the worst years of the epidemic and lack the perspectives of her older clients.

> A lot of my folks that struggle with adherence are very young, so they're not, you know, like HIV is not the death sentence that it once was. And they, like, you know, grew up in the same era that I did of thinking HIV is like no big deal now. Or maybe like, very shocked and surprised to get diagnosed and are living with a lot of shame and meds every day can contribute to that. (Paige)

Paige addressed that her older clients have had more time to process their emotions—grief, rage, confusion—that can accompany an HIV diagnosis, while her younger clients are still coming to terms with the reality of living with a chronic, incurable condition. Her reflections show an appreciation for how the trajectory and timing of the epidemic affects clients' experiences across generations, informing how she understands differences in medication adherence.

Participants expressed enthusiasm about recent developments in long-acting injectable medications, such as Cabenuva. Instead of having to take a pill every day, PLWHA now have the option to receive an injection once a month or every other month. Long-acting injectables hold great promise for PLWHA who struggle with pill fatigue, stigma, and issues such as substance use or unstable housing that contribute to poor adherence (Davis et al., 2024; Nachega et al., 2023; Trizzino et al., 2025). Participants observed increased acceptance and uptake of regimens like Cabenuva.

> Yeah, we have like 200 out of a thousand patients on Cabenuva. So it's been a big uptake and I think that has been, it doesn't, it's not necessarily a good option for everyone, but I think that that does make, create options for folks who do struggle with adherence or like, worry about their pills being found or have like, yeah, kind of a lot of instability in their life, just have being able to like, not have to worry about that goes a long way. (Tony)

Dan celebrated the rise of injectables. He noted that, in addition to the potential convenience and physical health benefits to this delivery method, there could also be psychological advantages as well.

> I do think injectables have offered a whole new kind of ballgame. Yeah, I think that was challenging because so much of treatment was, it felt very like symbolic of this thing that they were having difficulty understanding and I mean not to be annoying with metaphors but like swallowing or truly understanding things felt really hard. And so the act of like actively taking pills all the time was deeply traumatizing it seemed for a lot of folks…it feels very different than you come in, you get a shot, and then you're good for potentially months on end. So, yeah, I would say that felt like a pretty big shift just in terms of the shame or the reminders people feel like they're facing. (Dan)

Shame, the perceived sense that the self is somehow defective, contributes to suboptimal medication adherence and poor health outcomes (Bennett et al., 2016; Hutchinson & Dhairyawan, 2018; Walker, 2019). Dan's belief that injectables may alleviate shame around the virus and medications supports his belief that this delivery method may revolutionize HIV treatment.

For social workers who are not medical case managers, medication adherence was less relevant to their work with PLWHA. Josh, who provides psychotherapy to two PLWHA, noted that while he routinely asks clients about their use of psychotropic medications, he does not typically inquire about other medications, except for ART. For Josh, ART is something qualitatively different from other medications. When asked how they approach the issue of adherence with clients, Josh stated:

> None of my young clients are taking life-saving medication, unless it's their psych meds. You know, so this is where I think antiretrovirals are this weird middle-class medication, where it is like a life preserving medication and it's something we're talking about, it's in the room with us you know. And so it is this kind of thing I bring up that just is an easy way for me to just be like, oh yeah, you have HIV without saying, are you taking your meds every day? Are you feeling okay? Are your numbers low? Is everything in check? Yeah, there's easy ways to talk about it. Yeah, it's interesting to think about the overlap between the psychology of HIV and these medications, where it's like, I'm not going to ask my clients if they're taking their blood pressure medication. I don't ask my clients what they're taking. I don't want to know what they're taking. But this does impact their mental health in such an interesting way that it is like, I haven't really thought about that, in fact, I'm asking this client about a non-psych medication, pretty consistently. (Josh)

Josh's recognition that they ask their PLWHA clients about ART in ways that they would not with clients taking other life-preserving medication suggests that they consider HIV, despite the fact that the virus is now manageable, different or exceptional compared to other medical conditions. This theme will be more fully explored in Chapter 8.

Client Challenges and Barriers

Participants shared what they saw as the most common challenges and barriers experienced by their clients and how they responded to these challenges.

Client Challenges

The challenges experienced by clients can be grouped into three categories: health; material; and social. PLWHA live with a range of comorbidities that complicate their HIV care, including substance use and mental health concerns (Chhatre et al., 2021; Conway et al., 2021; Liu et al., 2024). As PLWHA populations grow older, clients exhibit health conditions normally associated with aging, which can further impede HIV care (Bennett et al., 2025; Martínez-Sanz et al., 2022; Thomas & Hoy, 2025). Substance use was the most frequently mentioned health concern. Nora shared how HIV and substance use often go hand in hand with her clients, impacting every facet of clients' wellbeing.

> It's sort of like I see it as sort of two pieces of string entwined together. And I don't know which comes first, you know, the HIV or the substance use. But yeah, it's prevalent, it's ever occurring. So you know, I think people try to go into treatment, but then they relapse because the supports don't exist to, you know, because of housing, because the rehab, the insurance only pays for so much for them to be in rehab, and as soon as they're released, they're back into the same settings that they were before. I've had patients lose their subsidized housing because they relapsed and, you know, that behavior sort of led to them losing their housing. (Nora)

For Nora, substance use cannot be understood as an isolated behavioral issue, but rather as a condition influenced by broader socioecological contexts. She viewed relapse as a consequence of unstable housing and restricted treatment options that place clients in precarious conditions that jeopardize recovery and HIV care.

Participants discussed the strategies they employ when working with clients who use substances. They returned to social work values and specific interventions meant to honor and uplift the voices of the individual client. Tony talked about how they use skills such as Motivational Interviewing (MI) and explore alternative treatment options to provide maximum choice to their clients.

> I use motivational interviewing and a harm reduction framework to talk about what their goals are, and also what the substances do or help them deal with, how is it helping them cope? Are there ways to shift that to another coping strategy if they want to and just kind of talking about how it functions for them and also providing support around safety, give out Narcan and talk with people about safer use practices in terms of not mixing drugs, using smaller amounts, not using alone. And then we also are able to offer medication-assisted treatment, making sure they understand those options and advocating with them with their provider. (Tony)

Tony's account demonstrates a socioecological approach to working with clients. The use of motivational interviewing and harm reduction techniques support the ethical principle of self-determination, while the advocacy with providers seeks to expand treatment access and choice.

In addition to substance use, participants addressed the prevalence of mental health disorders among their clients. Paige employed a socioecological model when discussing what she observes in her clients living with mental health challenges. In describing conditions with which her clients live, she suggested that systemic concerns such as poverty and violence contribute to poor mental health for her clients.

> I'm a social worker, so I really look at mental health and, you know, especially long-term mental health as like a person-in-environment, you know, as largely a product of what's going on, what's your background. Anxiety and depression are, you know, the most common, but I do see a lot of PTSD, a lot of our clients have been living in poverty or living as a disabled person for many, many years...And, you know, we do see some people on the schizophrenia spectrum, just a few though, really not too many. But I would say depression, anxiety, and PTSD are the big boys, so to speak. (Paige)

Paige leaned into her professional identity ("I'm a social worker") to explain how her approach to clients' mental health concerns diverges from that of other helping professionals, emphasizing a practice orientation that addresses the interactions between individual experiences and their social conditions.

Participants focused on a dearth of material resources and services that burden the lives of PLWHA. The paucity of affordable, safe, and consistent housing options was considered one of the most significant and challenging issues experienced by clients. Housing insecurity has been long recognized as a socioecological issue that contributes to substandard health and quality of life (Dombrowski et al., 2025; Dsouza et al., 2024; Liboro et al., 2024). Participants shared their exasperation at trying to locate suitable housing resources for their clients, noting that even with specialized programs for PLHWA, there are considerable gaps in the HIV safety net.

> Yes, housing is the biggest challenge that I would say people are experiencing,

> and the one that is the hardest to address. We do have a housing department…but it's always really tough to tell clients the way to get into that is to first be in the shelter system, because that's a really sucky way to have to get help and get subsidized housing. But that is often the biggest need that people come with. And sometimes people have kind of a misconception about case management or medical case management…can provide, thinking that they can come to case management and get access to housing. We do have some grants that we can like provide funds through to pay like first and last months' for moving or pay back rent and different things like that, pay utilities. But it's harder for folks who don't have any income at all. And that money wouldn't even really touch the surface. So housing, definitely. (Winnie)

Learning how to resolve client needs requires a socioecological perspective that allows social workers to navigate between individual-level factors of clients and structural constraints, a process central to professional identity formation as social workers come to understand the scope and limitations of their role.

Tony believed affordability was the central issue underlying the housing dilemma, pointing to policy-level dynamics that demonstrated a socioecological approach.

> But I think that, in my opinion, it's more about the systemic issues of affordability, like lack of rent control, lack of investment in affordable housing. And so even if, and a lack of tenant protections in general, so that people have like, more recourse. People struggle with housing because of the money piece, but also because they have to move because their building got sold or there has been a huge leak that was never fixed or some habitability issue that is not getting addressed. (Tony)

Their observation illustrate how economic policies and the absence of legal protections for renters expose PLWHA to housing insecurity that remains beyond their individual control.

Leo shared how housing insecurity can often be a lifelong challenge that predates clients' diagnoses. PLWHA often contend with complex life circumstances that can be difficult to resolve (Drew et al., 2020).

> Okay, there's folks who have never had their own stable housing because of income, because of, yeah, like substance use history or honestly just poverty…I had one individual who went through a divorce, got a leg amputation, was in the hospital and then in inpatient rehab, but then had nowhere to go after that and needed to find accessible housing like within a few weeks or else he'd be couch surfing but legless right, so that was a really unique situation but at the same time really hugely important that we help him. Yeah, yeah, I think that it's hard to describe exactly the issue, but I'll say a lot of our clients have had interesting lives that have taken them in many directions, and it's caused them to not have the stability that they need. And I think it's feeds into their whole life story of this, like, acquiring the virus, acquiring trauma, acquiring other issues. (Leo)

Leo's account illustrates that housing challenges are not just a matter of cost and availability but also reflect the personal history and identities that each client brings to the helping encounter.

Food insecurity was frequently mentioned as one of the more significant material challenges experienced by clients. PLWHA often struggle with meeting food expenses; food insecurity has negative effects on HIV care and overall wellbeing (Palar et al.,

2016; Tamargo et al., 2021; Tuthill et al., 2019). Even clients who receive food assistance find that such help is inadequate with rising grocery costs. Lynn acknowledged that in their city, there are specialized food banks that provide food for PLWHA, but they were conflicted by what they believed to be a lack of healthy offerings. They also shared how they work with clients to identify other resources in their area to supplement their personal pantries.

Participants stated clients do not always have reliable access to safe and affordable transportation. Transportation barriers decrease utilization of medical and social services among PLWHA (Pope et al., 2022; Sagrestano et al., 2014). Winnie shared that transportation services meant to get clients to their appointments can be widely inconsistent, frustrating both clients and social workers. Even when transportation is available, it may not be accessible for PLWHA with mobility issues. Paige stated that while they believed that public transportation options in their city were generally reliable, individuals who used walkers or wheelchairs were more limited in their options. Given the size of her city and the concentration of specialists in certain neighborhoods that were often far from clients' homes, Paige struggled to get her clients to important appointments due to limited transportation options for people with disabilities.

Participants observed that many of their clients experience social challenges such as loneliness. PLWHA, especially older adults, report that social isolation has negatively impacted their lives and health (Austin-Keiller et al., 2023; Pollak et al., 2025; Yoo-Jeong et al., 2020). Derek recalled his time facilitating a community space for PLWHA during his second-year practicum. He stated that for clients who participated in this resource, loneliness had a huge impact on their lives.

Yeah, I mean, there's a lot of stigma with the virus, and so internalizing that could be very complicated. I mean, a lot of issues for folks who are dating or having sex are around rejection, disclosure, not disclosing. Yeah, it really has an impact on one's self-image and maybe activates shame around some of the behavior that contributed to their diagnoses or anxieties and actual experience around rejection. It really contributes to a lot of avoidance socially, especially in contacts, romantic and sexual. So loneliness and HIV, I mean, are really, really huge. You know, there's of course a loneliness epidemic in general, but I think especially folks living with HIV and AIDS really struggle to feel, you know, like they belong and they can be loved. (Derek)

Derek adopted a socioecological approach in his conceptualization of clients' problems with loneliness. He did not portray loneliness as an individual-level issue, but as a consequence of a society that rejects and denies the relational and romantic needs of PLWHA. Collectively, these health, material, and social challenges highlight the complex and intersecting realities of PLWHA.

Reactions to Client Challenges

Participants were asked to reflect upon how they responded to clients experiencing challenges. Emma recalled a client with a long-term substance abuse problem. The client received referrals but would not engage in treatment. She shared how this served as a learning opportunity continues to inform her approach to social work.

I think, you know, it's easy to feel like, damn, what did I do this time? That maybe I didn't support this client the way I should have. But I think over the years I've learned that, like, my role isn't to help them. It's to guide them and empower them to help themselves. And that is all that I can do. And that is all that I can control.

> And that whatever I am there to support them with is only for their benefit. (Emma)

Emma turned to the ethical principle of self-determination to understand that behavior change ultimately lies with the client, a realization that helped her move beyond shame and guilt and toward greater clarity about the limits of her role.

Nora remembered a client with a lengthy history of mental health disorders and substance use and described their relationship as "abrasive". Over time, she would watch her client enter treatment and get well, only to relapse within days after discharge. While not an unusual occurrence in her line of work, Nora said clients like this weighed heavily upon her.

> I think it's challenging because it's not just her, then there are others, you know? It's sort of, yeah, it's layers that just sort of pile on top of each other. And every once in a while, you can peel one back, but more pile on than are taken off, I would say. (Nora)

Nora acknowledged there are clients she thinks about "constantly" because "I think there aren't enough systems to support" them. Nora's description of "layers" demonstrates how clients' challenges accumulate over time and across different domains of the socioecological model, often overwhelming available supports and discouraging early career social workers.

T discussed a client who consistently missed their doctor's appointments and failed to respond to repeated outreach. They used this situation to think critically about their approach to social work practice and the limitations of their role.

> It's a reminder to me that not everybody wants to take control of their life like

that. And it's good, it's a learning experience, as I always say. Everything's a learning experience. It's an opportunity to talk with my supervisor and see like, what can I be doing differently? Like, at what point do I decide that I'm doing my absolute best and I need to stop because they don't want to talk with me? They don't want to continue to engage with me. And it's a chance to like learn my limits, learn where I need to stop. Because I want to see him continue to be better. I want to see him continue to remain engaged in care because this patient is incredibly nice and incredibly sweet every time I talk to him. But he just doesn't want to remain engaged in care. He doesn't want to confront his status. (T)

As a student, T leaned into an educational opportunity. They shared how while they had a strong desire for their client to engage, they also understood that the client's wishes were paramount. For participants, observing their clients deal with health, material, and social challenges could be painful. These encounters revealed the impact of broader forces on their clients' lives while also serving as formative moments in their development as social workers. In these moments, as they engage with clients, they enact the values of the profession and learn what it means to be a social worker.

Client Strengths and Resources

Participants were also asked to identify their clients' strengths and resources. They also reflected upon their reactions to clients who successfully addressed their HIV care and other psychosocial stressors.

Client Strengths

Client strengths were divided into two categories, internal and external. Internal strengths are those positive attributes and capacities that exist within the individual client.

Participants frequently cited resilience as a strength of clients. Dulin and colleagues (2018), utilizing the socioecological model, define resilience as a set of positive psychological, behavioral, and/or social adaptations in the face of stressors and adversities. The protective and health-promoting aspects of resilience have a positive effect for PLWHA (Krause & Halkitis, 2024; Liboro et al., 2021; Meyers-Pantele et al., 2025). Ashley admired her clients' incredible fortitude in the face of difficult situations, but asserted they should not be subjected to obstacles that impede health and wellbeing.

> Like people are, I think, very resilient. And I think they understand a lot of the times that you can live a fairly normal life with HIV. And so I think that it takes an incredible amount of strength to have a chronic condition and then be like, I'm going to just function. Because I have chronic migraines. So it's not the same, but I go to work, and I interact with people. So having that connection of just being chronically ill, but also just rising above it and you know, just moving on, moving forward and just dealing with it is impressive. And it brings to mind resilience. And again, I hate that language because it shouldn't, you shouldn't have to be resilient. You know, there's just things that should be easy. (Ashley)

Resilience language can function to normalize systemic failures by shifting the burden of change onto an individual presumed to have the capacity and resources to adapt to adversity (Evans & Reid, 2015). Ashley was critical of discourses that valorize resilience yet leave intact the structural conditions that perpetuate hardships.

Participants noted the kindness and generosity they encountered when working with clients. Scott remembered that, despite the chaos and rigidity of the shelter system, many clients showed an incredible degree of patience.

> What most stood out to me was the kindness and forbearance that they showed to

> other people and to me. I think, yes, it's true that there can be a lot of violence and aggression on the street and in shelter…And at the same time, what I observed and experienced was a lot of patience and understanding. Patience and flexibility and understanding with rules, with changes in rules, with disruptions in shelter, with difficulties from new guests, with delays, with bad news, with plot twists in accessing resources, I found that by and large the clients, they understood that we were trying to help and that things did not always move in a straight line…It made me wonder how do people do that when they are going through life on the streets or in shelter and the stress of that, they're still making an effort to show respect and consideration. It was really incredible. (Scott)

Scott observed how clients would adjust to challenging situations with positive attitudes and understanding. The kindness that Scott experienced may be a way that clients foster and build their reserves of resilience (Sin, 2020; Slavich et al., 2022).

Participants felt that many clients had come to accept their HIV diagnosis and other stressors in their lives. Billy, a social worker with more than five years of post-MSW experience, shared how his clients remained grounded in the present and not stuck in wishful thinking, regrets, and reminiscences.

> I find that a lot of the individuals that I work with live in the moment. They're aware of this moment and being in this moment. And I think that's also part of the work that I was doing with individuals…was getting into this moment. Because there's nothing we can do about the woulda, shoulda, couldas. It's done. And there's nothing we can do about the what ifs. We have to be right now. We have to be in today. (Billy)

Living in regret has negative health consequences for PLWHA (Epstude & Jonas, 2015). For Billy's clients, living in the moment is not just a philosophy of life, but a necessary and practical survival technique.

External strengths are the resources and supports clients employ in their interactions with the world. Self-advocacy, the ability to recognize and assert one's needs and influence decisions, was noted as a primary external strength. PLWHA who engage in self-advocacy may experience better health outcomes and more positive encounters with treatment providers (Brashers et al., 2002; Brashers et al., 2006). Winnie shared their appreciation for clients who continue to self-advocate in spite of indifferent or inadequate systems of care.

> Clients can be really amazing advocates for themselves. Like it's, it's really phenomenal. Especially some clients who have really been through the ringer, they do not stop being advocates for themselves. And, you know, speaking up when they don't feel they are getting fair service, speaking up when they have needs, you know, asking to speak to a supervisor if they need extra assistance. I really admire that because, yeah, a lot of times I think people can be afraid to ask for help or feel ashamed of that. And then they kind of slip into the background and it's easy for case managers to think, oh, this person's not reaching out and so they have low needs and so I don't need to reach out, so it's fine. And I've definitely kind of seen a few instances of that happening. And so it is really nice when clients can just continue to be their self-advocate. (Winnie)

Winnie revealed that self-advocacy can be an essential response to systems that overlook or underestimate individuals who do not actively assert their needs. What is often framed as an individual virtue can also be understood as evidence of systemic failure.

Participants also discussed that many clients had high levels of health literacy and positive engagement with treatment providers. PLWHA who demonstrate good health literacy have been found to have better HIV care outcomes (Mgbako et al., 2022; Wawrzyniak et al., 2013). August respected that clients, many of whom were dealing with multiple challenges, were active participants in their health care.

> Their dedication to their health and to making sure that they were on top of their viral load and CD4 counts were honestly remarkable. I often thought about if I were in a similar situation, my meds would honestly be like a lot…their level of self-care around their health was pretty remarkable to me. They understood that if they did not take care of their health there was no possibility to survive if they were experiencing some pretty severe homelessness or any type of housing. (August)

The strengths demonstrated by clients enable more sustained engagement with social workers and other systems of care, even in the context of significant hardships. Client strengths are not merely worthy qualities, but practical resources that supported continuity of care and the ongoing formation of relationships.

Reactions to Client Strengths

Participants discussed some of their success stories in working with PLWHA and how they were impacted by these encounters. Dan recalled a client who struggled with their gender identity and later identified as transgender. He shared how happy he was to be part of his client's journey.

> I mean, it's really meaningful. I mean, I feel self-aware while saying this, because I feel like this is almost a cliché of people being in this space, but I do feel privileged to be part of some of this…I think being able to be in a clinical setting where work is being done that seems meaningful and grounded and thoughtful and to see, yeah, patients who are able to find stability and find self and, you know, in whatever various biopsychosocial measures do well. I mean, that's a really exciting thing. So yeah, for me, it's a, not to overstate, but it's been an honor at times. Like, it really can be a nice thing. (Dan)

For Dan, the clinical setting was more than a site of service delivery; it was a space where meaningful, relational work with clients could occur. These environments can nurture clients' wellbeing and sustain social workers who derive purpose from the work, enhancing their professional development. In the next chapter, I examine the organizational-level factors that cultivate supportive settings where both clients and social workers can thrive.

Vanessa shared about her work with a Deaf client who had difficulties maintaining a residence due to a lack of life skills and living in unsafe neighborhoods. Her client qualified for temporary housing and they worked together to address issues such as budgeting and paying bills. Vanessa learned some rudimentary American Sign Language (ASL) to improve her communication with the client. She related how this work made her grateful.

> It makes you reflect on what you, your day-to-day struggles and think about theirs. It kind of humbles you a little bit. It makes you just think about what you need to be grateful for. It also makes me want to do better for my patients. Like, I started taking ASL classes so I can better communicate with them. When I

first met him, I couldn't do any. I was like, hi, like I was very limited. I felt so bad not being able to communicate with him to the point where I was like, okay, I have to fix this because I don't like feeling like I can't communicate with him. It just made me like, overall, I want to push myself to do better. So that way it could help other people too in the long run. (Vanessa)

By observing her client demonstrate capacity from growth and change, Vanessa was inspired to learn a new skill that she could use with this client and Deaf and/or hard-of-hearing clients in the future. She expanded her practice skills and responsiveness to client needs, a process that contributed to her ongoing professional development and the ethical principle of competence. Vanessa's observations of her client's willingness to change inspired her own change behaviors.

Jenny was assigned to work with a client whom she initially struggled to develop a rapport. Her client believed that she was keeping housing resources from him,and he would complain to her supervisor about what he perceived to be a lack of effort on Jenny's part. Eventually they were able to repair their relationship, and Jenny found a space for her client in a new housing program suitable for his needs. Her client was very thankful for all of Jenny's work. Reflecting upon this experience, Jenny said the work motivated her but also made her more aware of her own limitations as a social worker.

I think it's really reinforcing because I think that for some of my clients there's things that I have no control of. You know a lot of people need housing, they need a job, they need food and if it were up to me, I would give you the house. I would give you the food, I would give you everything you need. Unfortunately, this is not up to me. And when you know I get positive feedback or I'm able to help someone it really does feel good and I think it reminds me of why I got into social

> work because there are people who unfortunately don't have all the basic necessities that they need. And so, you know, it just keeps me motivated to continue to help my clients and continue to seek out resources that can be useful to my clients and to other people. (Jenny)

As her client modeled resilience, Jenny developed her own professional resilience that continues to support her social work practice. Witnessing client strengths and hard-fought accomplishments within complex socioecological environments encouraged participants to expand their ideas of what is possible for clients to achieve, which is an important developmental task in the lives of early career social workers.

The Role of Relationship

Relationship is fundamental to social work practice (Dix et al., 2025; Howe et al., 2018). The NASW Code of Ethics (2021) highlights the importance of human relationships as one of the six ethical principles of the profession. Participants shared how relationship factored into their work with PLWHA. Several participants discussed the need to develop appropriate boundaries with clients as an intervention that encourages self-sufficiency and responsibility. Nora expressed her frustrations working with clients whose expectations do not align with her social work role.

> I've been thinking about this a lot lately. I'm feeling maybe some signs of burnout because our work is so relational that I go home with my clients, in a sense, you know, they sort of live it inside my head. But I guess with clients, I'm willing to do the work as much as you're willing to do. I cannot do more than you are willing to do to help you. I try to make that clear. I try to have boundaries just for myself. I'm available 9 to 5, you know, Monday through Friday. And I'm happy to,

> if you ask me for something that maybe is not really what I do as a medical case manager, I'm happy to do it if you're here doing it with me, but I'm not just going to go and do it off on my own. I guess I don't know. I want them to know that I'm here to support them, but only if they're also here, if that makes sense. (Nora)

Nora spoke to the toil her work has on her wellbeing. Although central to social work practice, relational demands upon social workers incur costs, including burnout, that are especially injurious for early career social workers who may be overwhelmed with their responsibilities and lacking sufficient supports (Cleece et al., 2025). Paige emphasized her desire for clients to become more involved in the helping relationship.

> I just give them the information that they need and kind of leave it up to them. I come from, I'm very much like, you know, I can't care about this more than you do. And also, this is your thing. If you want to make it happen, I will go so hard for you, but I am not going to work harder on this than you are willing to care about it, right? (Paige)

This statement reveals a professional orientation that prioritizes mutual engagement and self-determination. For early career social workers, this position represents an effort to balance client wellbeing with an understanding that change must be internally motivated rather than externally imposed.

Ashley also stressed the role of accountability and client empowerment in her work. She recalled how her methods conflicted with medical providers with her organization, who she believed inappropriately enabled clients.

> I lean more towards the, you can do this yourself kind of person and not because I don't want to do things, but because I think it empowers people, and I might not

> be around to do it...One of the biggest issues in our clinic right now is that our providers will continue prescribing for patients who don't show for their appointments. They continue to refill. And I, I'm like, I have never seen anything like this in my entire life, but they're like, oh, we don't want them to spread it. And I'm like, people have agency…We have people who haven't been seen in like two years who are getting refills. And they're like, oh, I feel ethically bound to do that because it's not like diabetes where it's just a you problem, like you can spread it. And I was like, yeah, but you're talking about people as if they're sex machines. You have the choice to use protection. Your partner has the choice to go on PrEP and use a condom. So obviously I do, I move with compassion, but also like, I try to assume the best of people's agency and try to empower people. (Ashley)

Ashley demonstrated that expectations of personal accountability were not incompatible with compassionate approaches to client care, but rather an essential component of support aligned with the ethical principles of the profession.

Jenny acknowledged her ideas about relationship in social work have changed over the course of her emerging career. She discovered she is more effective when she takes time to know her clients better and establish trust, which encourages collaborative engagement.

> I think that as a new social worker, I initially viewed the client and social work relationship as, you're coming in with something, with a problem, and I need to find a solution to help you. And over the years, now that I have a little bit more of experience, I've found that I now like to get to know the person more, have a more relaxed conversation...And so, you know, really having a conversation or building that relationship with this person so that they don't feel there's a certain dynamic

that's going on, that you're above them because you are in a helping position. But yeah, I think it's really important to have a good relationship with your clients. Sometimes people don't disclose certain things to you that are crucial to their care because they don't trust you. And so really, like slowly building that relationship with people will really get you to a point where they trust you and you're able to really support them in any way you can. (Jenny)

Jenny understood the significance of relationship as a condition that supports clients' goal achievement (Walsh, 2021). For PLWHA who often hold multiple stigmatized identities and have received substandard help from systems of care, a strong working relationship is especially crucial (Shernoff, 2014). Jenny's reflection demonstrates how early career social workers refine their understanding of practice over time, as repeated encounters with clients prompt a reconsideration of previously held assumptions about the helping relationship.

Dan emphasized that in his work as a behavioral health consultant for PLWHA, relationship plays an essential role. He downplayed the selection of modalities and specific interventions and concentrated on the close connections he creates with clients. Factors outside the technical components of therapy, such as the quality of the working relationship, may explain more of client change than the specific form of therapy provided (Cameron, 2014; Drisko, 2013).

But yeah, for most of my patients, I'm not really doing impressive interventions...Most of the work is literally just showing up and in an appropriate capacity, like loving on our patients. It's really just the, however you want to word that, the way that sounds more appropriate. But it's really, it's about, yeah, it's about love. It's about these deep connections. And it's obviously only done in a professional clinical capacity, but it's just a really warm caring space where our doctors have worked with patients for their entire lives...I would say relationships are like the integral component of the work we do...That really feels like the priority in the clinic. (Dan)

Dan noted that because of the now-chronic nature of HIV, his clients often have a consistent and long-standing presence in the clinic, creating opportunities to develop more enduring relationships with social workers and other providers. This sustained engagement allows for early career social workers to deepen their understanding of their clients' experiences, observe how multiple systems impact clients, and strengthen their emerging professional identity.

Issa identified a challenge they encountered in creating relationship with PLWHA clients. They were drawn to their practicum site because of the organization's long-standing history of working with queer communities, with which Issa identifies.
However, they recognized that their queer identity was vastly different from their clients.

> A lot of my interest is in working with the queer community...and how even though I'm queer, my queer experience felt so far from mostly these gay men who were a handful of decades older than me, and their very specific experience, the HIV/AIDS epidemic, and so much of that feels like a very specific subculture within a broader queer community. I think maybe even less so the diagnosis itself and more so the cultural knowledge around it felt like there was a distance, that maybe they didn't expect me to understand...I had a close friend who's a young White gay man and I felt like maybe even he was more expected to understand, and they saw him and they felt more like, oh yeah, you're part of us. (Issa)

While shared identities and experiences between client and social worker may facilitate a helping relationship, they are not sufficient (Bishop et al., 2022). Issa's experience illuminates how generational location within the epidemic informs the meanings attached to HIV and queer identities, which in turn influence the expectations and dynamics of the helping relationship.

Derek, who lives with HIV, believed his serostatus offered him insight into the experiences of his PLWHA clients. However, he understood that identities and experiences beyond a shared diagnosis might complicate the helping relationship.

> I have a lot of history living with HIV and AIDS, but a lot of my experience was around gay culture and HIV and AIDS and that whole history and how important it is but encountering folks living with HIV who weren't gay and also weren't White, there wasn't a sort of cultural lineage, it was more...I don't know what word to use, but like ego alien or something. And not having the same sense of possible cultural social identification made it that much harder to sort of internalize it or claim it as like a part of their identity in a positive way. (Derek)

Derek use of "ego alien" may refer to ego-dystonicity, suggesting that his clients' experiences of HIV did not mesh with his interpretation of the epidemic. The absence of reference points made the helping relationship more complex than he anticipated. The meanings Derek developed around HIV were shaped by the historical and cultural contexts in which he encountered the epidemic, particularly within White gay communities. As one of the oldest participants, his more extensive engagement with HIV afforded him a perspective on the epidemic that contrasted with younger participants who experienced a different era.

Generational Differences in Client Cohorts

As HIV approaches its sixth decade, there is increasing diversity in age among PLWHA. Participants shared their thoughts about generational differences between their clients. They discussed two distinct cohorts: younger PLWHA, usually considered under 30 years of age, who were more recently diagnosed; and older adults above the age of 50 who have been living with the virus for decades. While this binary construction proved heuristically appealing, it collapses the heterogeneity of PLWHA and obscures important nuances. While older PLWHA, defined as individuals aged 50 and older (Sankar et al., 2011), have the lowest rates of new infections, there was a 15% increase in incidence in this age group from 2015 to 2019; this was the largest increase among all age groups (Justice et al., 2022; Russell & Justice, 2024). Older adults who are newly diagnosed have been described as a forgotten population (Ellman et al., 2014). Branas and colleagues (2022) examined the health outcomes of older PLWHA and stratified them into two groups: long-term survivors (individuals diagnosed before 1996, when ART was introduced); and individuals diagnosed after 1996. Long-term survivors had higher rates of comorbid complications, including greater prevalence of cancer, COPD, osteoarthritis, and psychological disorders, in conjunction with lower quality of life when compared to older PLWHA diagnosed after 1996. Within both cohorts, there are considerable variations in race, ethnicity, sexual orientation, and gender identity and expression, among other identities (Brennan et al., 2013; Gabriel et al., 2023).

Participants described how their approaches to practice varied in response to the generational cohort of their clients. Paige viewed her older clients as more reliant on case management on a long-term basis, while younger clients required more help to become self-sufficient and ultimately discharged from case management.

And, you know, I have two age groups of clients, the folks that have been living with the AIDS epidemic that are like Gen Xers or Boomers. I have people that are, you know, they are more like aunties or even like parents to me that I just, I check in on them, I make sure they're doing good, get them set up with home healthcare when they need it. And then I have people that are more like my age, and we joke at work that that's just kind of like chatting with the girls, you know, just like connecting...A lot of them are living with addiction. And so you can't pay your rent, like, here's what's available to you or, and really with that group, it's teaching them how to like be adults, be responsible adults, and helping them attain stability so that they can kind of graduate from case management and that they don't need a point person, they can figure it out on their own. Where my survivors of the AIDS epidemic, that's not really a realistic goal for them. It's more about helping them as they age with HIV. (Paige)

Paige, a Millennial, identified her older clients as "aunties" and "parents", suggesting that she sees her social work role almost as a caretaker function. However, she views her younger clients more like peers ("chatting with the girls") with whom she is working on developing skills to support independence. Paige's differing perspectives of each cohort appear to shape her expectations for her clients and the strategies she employs in her work with them.

According to August, older adults who have interacted with systems of care for many years hunger for meaningful connections with their treatment providers and social workers, while younger PLWHA assume a more transactional approach.

I think the older folks who have been living with HIV for much longer than the youth I was working with, I think that they had a profound sense of, if I trust you

> with this, you're my people and...there was almost like a reverence, I think, for relationship and connection, in more of the context of providing care as a care provider, for maybe my role as a clinician. As for youth, they are kind of coming to the clinic and just expecting to get a service and then leave. Whereas I think some of the older clients or patients that I've worked with want to establish an actual relationship with me, with their doctor, with their case manager, any person that they're interacting with. They don't just want to show up and feel like that person is extracting information from them because they need it for Medicare or Medicaid or something. They want to actually know you because they're going to be interfacing with this system and engaging in the system for their life. (August)

August shared that his younger clients were learning how to adapt to their diagnosis, especially relating to dating, sex, and issues of confidentiality. He believed his older adults were more likely to have achieved a "level of self-actualization" and made meaning of their experiences living with HIV. Like Paige, August's interpretations of generational differences influenced how he tailored his social work practice across cohorts.

Billy believed that most organizations were ill-equipped to meet the needs of older PLWHA. He remembered hearing from older PLWHA who visited a well-known organization in his city to receive services. These clients reported that younger staff members could not communicate with or relate to older individuals. Billy said older PLWHA "didn't feel like they were being seen". Organizations that provide medical care and social services to PLWHA often have gaps in their programming that minimize and exclude older PLWHA (Cox & Brennan-Ing, 2017; Wallach & Brotman, 2019). Billy's observations carried particular weight as the oldest participant, drawing upon his longstanding personal and community connections to the epidemic. He was attuned to the challenges of older PLWHA in ways not reflected in the accounts of younger participants.

In his work providing psychotherapy to a younger adult living with HIV, Josh stated their client had no knowledge of the history of HIV. Josh, one of the older participants, remembered how they would hear the stories from their friends who almost died because of the virus; their associations with PLWHA were unlike that of any of the younger participants. They provided their client resources and information about the virus but doubted the client engaged with the material.

> I don't think they...they do not have this perspective at all. And I'm not going to shove it down their throat. I think I told them to watch at one point *How to Survive a Plague*, which is one of the documentaries that came out about ACT UP. But I don't know what they did. (Josh)

While Josh believed an appreciation of the history of HIV is important, they recognized the limitations of their role. Even when describing different interactions with clients, participants generally acknowledged that generational differences influenced their approach to practice.

Salience of HIV in the Lives of Clients

Participants discussed their beliefs about the salience of HIV in the lives of clients. As HIV has shifted to a chronic, manageable condition, the virus has become less prominent in public discourse (Linnemayr, 2015). While HIV has been shown to contribute to a person's sense of self and identity (Sematlane et al., 2024), concerns such as poverty and unemployment may take greater precedence (Justesen, 2011). Overwhelmingly, participants revealed they felt that HIV was not considered the main problem, or even a problem at all, in clients' lives. Participants related that material challenges, those factors that make daily living burdensome, were more intractable than the virus. Paige vividly remembered her work with a long-time client of her organization who began to display unruly behavior onsite, including yelling at staff and urinating on the floors. During a case consultation with the client's medical team and other providers, she said that, for this client, HIV was not the issue.

> And during those meetings, I remember saying HIV is actually the least of my concerns. His labs are excellent. And that rings true for many of my clients that, especially my older clients, have been living with HIV for my entire lifetime. Their HIV is well managed. Their finances, however, are, you know, a different story. Mental health is a different story. And even with my younger clients, I don't know if it is as a society, we like to see HIV, HIV is no longer a big deal. But yeah, HIV tends to be really not a primary concern for most people, unless they're newly diagnosed, and then, of course, they're still grappling with all the feelings around their diagnosis. But once they've had it for even a couple of years, they're just like, okay, whatever. (Paige)

Paige's account reflects how social workers make meaning of HIV at this point in the epidemic, not as an isolated medical issue, but as one element of a broader and often more urgent set of socioecological challenges affecting clients' lives.

Other participants concurred with Paige's belief that HIV is "no longer a big deal". Scott stated his initial attitudes and beliefs about HIV were formed during his adolescence. However, biomedical progress has prioritized material concerns, such as housing and food security, over HIV health.

> It [HIV] seemed incidental in the sense that when I would ask someone or talk

with someone about the circumstances and what are we going to deal with together, how are we going to try to resolve your housing crisis, it was just one of many other variables to take into consideration. And it was not the most immediate one in our face. The one that was biggest, most immediate in our face was this person has been living on the street. They may have no clothing. They may not have consistent access to a bathroom. They may be hungry. They may be experiencing symptoms of mental illness. They may also have a substance use disorder. And oh, by the way, they also have HIV, but it's generally stable, generally under control…it was very easy to say, okay, they had HIV, yes, but there are some bigger issues that are taking precedence right now, which felt almost counterintuitive to the impression I had gotten growing up, which is that HIV is the biggest and the baddest of them all. And then here in this situation, it really was not. It was not the biggest and the baddest. It was, oh yeah, that, you know, that too, add it to the list. (Scott)

Scott situated the virus and his clients' presenting problems within a larger matrix of social, structural, and temporal contexts that initially challenged his preconceptions about the virus. In the next chapter, I explore how social workers come to see their clients' diagnosis not as a barrier, but as a pathway to specialized services and benefits.

Josh shared that even though their two psychotherapy clients living with HIV may not explicitly address their serostatus, it still has a presence in the clinical space. Josh compared their experiences working with these clients to their work with queer and trans clients who may not want to talk about issues of sexual orientation or gender identity and expression.

Honestly, it's not I mean, the thing is, neither of my clients are like, that's the that's

> the focus of our work. It's so interesting...I have so many queer clients or trans clients who like don't want to talk about being queer or trans or, but it's like, it is a thread in the weave of our therapy, but they don't want that to be the focus. And I would say this is kind of a similar thing where we're never, neither of my clients were never specifically talking about this as an issue, but we are, it just slips in inevitably about how it impacts them having sex or whether or not they tell their friends or whether or not they, you know, but they're not coming in being like, oh, yeah, we need to talk about my HIV diagnosis again. You know, which is different because I feel some part of me is like, let's talk, let's Gestalt it, just give it the chair in the room with us. We don't have to talk to it all the time, but it's there...And I think they would rather let it present itself when it needs to. (Josh)

For Josh's clients, HIV is a background presence in their lives, even when it is not openly addressed in therapy. Informed by their prior experiences with PLWHA, Josh expressed a desire to give HIV a "chair" in the room, while remaining attuned to their clients' readiness to engage with it.

Self-Disclosure with PLWHA

Self-disclosure is widely regarded as one of the more complex and contested practices within social work. Knight (2012) distinguishes between two types of self-disclosure: self-revealing, where the social worker shares their thoughts and reactions about the work with the client; and self-involving, where the social worker offers experiences from their life outside of the helping relationship. Participants were questioned about their uses of self-disclosure with PLWHA and what lessons they received about self-disclosure during their social work education and practicums. They were also asked whether they ever disclosed their own serostatus to clients. Participants were instructed they were not expected to disclose their serostatus; however, most participants shared this information.

Most examples of self-disclosure offered by participants qualified as self-involving. One of the more common disclosures involved participants' past use of substances. Disclosure felt particularly important for Luca in their work with individuals with substance use concerns. They believed self-disclosure enhanced the helping relationship.

> My substance use experiences were different than many of the folks that I supported at the exchange, but there were definite overlaps that I could connect with, and I think that they could connect with me too, that it felt I could provide a different form of empathetic care because I had some of those shared experiences that many other folks in my cohort did not... In the syringe exchange, people would ask...if I used before, if I'd injected before, and all sorts of questions. Yeah, and I wouldn't go into great detail, but I would usually tell them that, yeah, that I had used in the past and that I was, yeah, like five years sober. (Luca)

Social workers who use self-disclosure must negotiate tensions around boundaries, ethics, and the use of self, which can be daunting for even the most experienced practitioners. Luca, who was in their first-year practicum, demonstrated how they worked through these issues in practice by balancing what they comfortable sharing and what needed to remain private.

Participants shared a range of their lived experiences and identities to clients. Paige disclosed her use of psychotropic medications. She used that experience to assist clients who have problems with consistent medication adherence. Paige shared how she uses self-disclosure as a form of psychoeducation.

> If it's somebody that's just younger and they're just having trouble being a stable person, I can relate to that. And I really try to approach them from a stance of like, you know, I get it. And I use my role to keep myself accountable. Like, I don't miss my SSRIs because how can I be preaching to my clients if I'm not doing it? Right. We try to identify, is there somebody in your life that you talk to every day? OK, maybe when you're FaceTiming them, you can take your meds while you're on the phone with them. And they know or, you know, I use an app to keep track of my meds. So here's the app I use. Try this. (Paige)

Paige's account demonstrates that medication adherence is not simply a matter of individual responsibility, but one that can be supported through relational interventions and the introduction of accountability routines and social connections.

In Jenny's work with Latino clients, she disclosed her shared ethnic identity to create connections with clients who come from communities that hold stigmatized beliefs about sexual orientation and HIV. She believed that her background offered insight into clients' fears and facilitated the helping relationship. In her words, "[t]his is when I can empathize with them and really get to that level of explaining to them that it's not their fault that they are not able to do this, or they're not able to have good relationships with their family members. It's a lot of generational curses that you were taught when you were a kid. Like, you know, that men should only marry women and women should only marry men". Jenny used self-disclosure to convey empathy while helping clients make sense of their experiences within larger socioecological contexts. The accounts of Luca, Paige, and Jenny reveal that self-disclosure is a dynamic and context-dependent practice.

As early career social workers, decisions about whether and how to self-disclose become part of their emerging professional identity as they learn how to integrate their experiences into social work practice.

August shared that he self-disclosed more often in his work with PLWHA compared to other client populations. He believed that deeper emotional engagement was necessary in response to the challenges experienced by PLWHA.

> I feel in that work I self-disclosed more to my clients just about anything, about my life or how I was feeling about our relationship between me and the client. Because it felt important to do that. Because there were so much vulnerability and information...there had to be so much you got to know people on a super deep level like their daily, like knew exactly what time they woke up and what their morning routine was, you just got to know so much about them that I think it was only fair that they could be in your life a little bit in some way…that doesn't mean that you're meeting them outside of work, but it means that there's a little bit more reciprocity in the relationship...I feel like I bring more of my entire self or need to do that when I'm working with clients with HIV, if that makes sense. (August

August's experience reinforces the idea that social work with PLWHA requires an approach to practice that goes beyond conventional uses of self-disclosure. He believed HIV involves unique circumstances that necessitated different types of interventions, a theme that is explored in more detail in Chapter 8.

Other participants challenged the need for self-disclosure. Scott shared he did not believe self-disclosure was necessary in his work and that his effectiveness could be maintained through the use of strong boundaries with his clients.

> I never self-disclosed at any point and that was purposeful and that was something that I felt clear about that it is…it felt like it was not necessary, was simply not necessary to the work. It wasn't necessary to establish rapport to establish trust, and it would not have added anything, in my opinion. It just wasn't necessary. And it was part of my effort to maintain boundaries as well. (Scott)

When asked whether she uses self-disclosure in her work, Nora said that she had a similar approach to Scott.

> Not often. Not often. I'm someone who in conversation likes to turn around and talk about the other person. I'll just start asking questions. And maybe my job has made me good at that. I do get clients that will say, I love you, and I'm not someone who easily reciprocates that language. So, you know, I'll find words to say where I don't have to sort of be vulnerable in those moments. But yeah, I've gotten good at it. I'm flexing that muscle for myself. (Nora)

Nora desired some protection and distance from her clients. Vulnerability was framed as something to be avoided, and this avoidance has become a skill in Nora's social work armamentarium. There is little instruction in practice skills and no clear guidelines to support social workers in deciding how and when to make effective and ethical self-disclosures (McDonnell & Wayland, 2024). Early career social workers, who encounter dilemmas about self-disclosure without the supports available in their MSW programs or consistent on-the-job supervision, may find these situations even more challenging.

Lessons About Self-Disclosure

Participants were asked what they learned about self-disclosure during the course of their social work studies and practicum experiences. Luca remembered that their MSW program suggested limited uses of self-disclosure, but they found this messaging incompatible with their experiences in practicum.

> I think one area, and this continues to be a challenging piece, was around the self-disclosure. And at the time, when I was in my MSW program, there was still a lot of conversation about, like, essentially disclose as little as possible, was what was shared. And I'm like, okay, cool...but I think it felt more important with the humans I was working with to share a little bit more, to be a little bit more human with them. I think that many of them had had a lot of interactions with providers especially that felt really distanced and felt like kind of cold and like disconnected...And that, I think, continues to be a challenge. How do we navigate disclosure in a way that allows us to be authentic humans with people but also be mindful of what that kind of disclosure can do to a working alliance? (Luca)

Luca described their use of self-disclosure as a way to repair rupture their clients experienced from providers who lacked personal awareness of the challenges of substance use. Luca identified that what they learned in the classroom was contrary to what they were experienced with clients. For early career social workers, resolving such tensions is an important professional developmental task.

Jenny remembered what she was taught in her program and stated that she is developing her own approach to self-disclosure.

> Well, during my social work studies, they always mentioned like disclosing personal information. And they mentioned it to be limited. They always said that to really watch out what you're disclosing to your client because it may be triggering to them as well. And for also the safety of them and myself as well. But

> I always was like, had this like really big barrier to never saying anything about my personal life because of how they may interpret it or how they may see me as a professional. So yeah…I have slowly been disclosing when appropriate. Little details, but nothing major. (Jenny)

Like Luca, Jenny described a disconnect between how self-disclosure was taught and the realities of her practice. As she grew more comfortable in her role, she was increasingly confident in using self-disclosure in an appropriate manner. This growth demonstrates the growth of a professional identity formation that seeks to incorporate both formal learning and practice experience.

From the outset of his studies, Scott said he was "very strict about self-disclosure…I do not see it as necessary". Scott had many years of working in social services prior to his MSW studies and found that he could be effective in his role without self-disclosure. He believed his program gave contradictory messaging around self-disclosure.

> I think social work education took a different approach where it seems like there was a lot of emphasis placed on tell your story, tell who you are, tell me your identity, tell me more, tell me more, tell me more, and I didn't like that. I think the approach was, we have to tell you clinically that self-disclosure should be strategic, but we are going to celebrate disclosure when it happens, and I didn't particularly resonate with that. I didn't find that helpful or healthy for me. (Scott)

In her study of social workers' attitudes and experiences with self-disclosure, Knight (2012) found that half of the respondents disagreed that their education prepared them to engage in self-disclosure, while over 60% stated that they disagreed that they felt comfortable seeking guidance from a supervisor or colleague regarding self-disclosure. Participants' accounts suggest that self-disclosure is a significant concern for most early career social workers, pointing to a need for more comprehensive instruction in classrooms and practicums.

Self-Disclosure of HIV Status

Participants were asked whether clients inquired about their HIV status and how they responded. Most participants did not experience such questions but some recounted how they addressed this issue. August believed that these questions were to be expected and compared such queries to those he received regarding his sexual orientation.

> I think that was a fair question for them to want to know. It's the same question that I feel I get from when I'm talking with a new client in my private practice who wants to work with me. They want to know if I'm queer, because that's really important that they have a queer affirming therapist, or if somebody has a lived experience, just knowing. So I would, yeah, I would tell them I am not positive, but I have been, this has been my career, has been, even though it's not been long, but like it's my entire career has been focused on, all my energy has been focused on working with folks living with HIV, and I'm very passionate and dedicated to this and that's how I would communicate that. (August)

For August, self-disclosure served as a way to reassure clients that he understood HIV and its challenges and that his commitment to working with PLWHA did not depend on sharing their serostatus.

Billy self-disclosed his long history and engagement with PLWHA and HIV activism to demonstrate to clients he was aware of their challenges despite being HIV-negative.

> I was asked those questions by clients, and I did share my status with clients when they would ask. And, you know, I'm HIV negative…but I've also shared with them how, you know, how many people I lost and why I'm negative, you know, but also that fear, sharing that first test. It took two weeks to get your results, the first time I had an HIV test. And I was convinced I was dying. I was so sure I had HIV. Because I was just as big a slut as all my friends, you know. I was just as big a trashy slut as they were, and it didn't happen to me. (Billy)

Billy drew upon his personal experiences and historical understanding of the virus to inform his use of self-disclosure, in a way that August, who is three decades younger than Billy, could not. While self-disclosure often functions to highlight common ground between social worker and client, August and Billy demonstrated that, even without the lived experience of HIV, their personal and professional backgrounds provided insight that guided their work.

Derek was the only participant to disclose that he is living with HIV; he also shared that he has a history of past substance abuse. He worked with PLWHA during both of his MSW practicums. In his second year, Derek worked for an organization that hosted a drop-in center for PLWHA who were also living with mental health concerns. He remembered how he worked closely with his supervisor to develop his approach to self-disclosure and explained why it felt appropriate in this setting.

> I think especially around HIV because it's such a stigmatized disease and it's, you know, sort of comorbid with feelings of alienation and loneliness that it felt really important for me to disclose pretty immediately…I did talk in supervision quite a bit

about that choice…I decided to do it and the community members, some of them had been there for two decades, so they never had a staff member who disclosed their lived experience, you know. And that was really special to me, because some of them had been there for, you know, like two decades and had seen Lord knows how many staff members. So, for someone in that role, to sort of bridge that gap and let them know their shared experience was very moving for me, hopefully for them. I imagine, I don't know. (Derek)

At a formative moment in his professional development, Derek turned to supervision to guide his use of self-disclosure. Despite finding the practice meaningful, he remained uncertain about how sharing his serostatus affected the working relationship. Clients may perceive self-disclosing helping professionals as more authentic, but injudicious uses of self-disclosure without attention to important contextual factors can potentially disrupt the work (Audet & Everall, 2010; Robertson et al., 2025).

As Derek has gained more social work experience, he has been more discriminating in disclosing his HIV status. His account suggest professional maturation, in which early reliance on self-disclosure shifts to a more nuanced approach informed by deeper clinical judgment.

> Anyways, as I become more sort of confident in my general sort of clinical abilities, I do question a bit, okay, my idea was I'm doing it for them to sort of allow identification, make them feel less alone, make them feel understood. But I also understood I was gratifying something about me, which is, you know, okay, I guess. To be a bit more cautious about that and be more mindful. I'm less quick to disclose my HIV status or that I'm in recovery with folks than I was initially. I mean, I think the relationship itself can be healing. Yeah. Over time though, I have

been a bit more guarded and cautious about self-disclosure. (Derek)

Derek was also concerned that colleagues might question his use of self-disclosure. Weighing the pros and cons, he believed that "because of my history of activism…it's important for me to name it". His use of self-disclosure is not merely an intrapsychic debate, but a careful decision informed by the confluence of personal experience and socioecological factors.

Conclusion

Interpersonal factors that address the relationships between the social work and their client affect the effectiveness of social work interventions. In this chapter, participants shared how they were able to cultivate rapport, empathy, and collaboration with their clients, sometimes in difficult situations. The recognition of these interpersonal factors within the socioecological model is critical to ensure that social work practice with PLWHA remain grounded in the relational values of the profession.

Chapter 6

Organizational-Level HIV Service Environments

The organizational factors within the socioecological model consist of policies, practices, cultures, and conditions of the agencies and institutions established to empower and care for PLWHA. Through an analysis of factors such as leadership, collaboration with colleagues, and workplace climate, social workers can better understand how organizations support and/or constrain their efforts on behalf of clients. Eight themes emerged from the data: social workers' interest in their organization; responsibilities of their employment; satisfaction with their employment; experiences with supervision; intra-organization collaboration; organizational benefits of HIV diagnosis; role of the organization in the lives of clients; and organizational responses to current events.

Interest in the Organization

Several participants reported they selected their place of employment and/or practicum site specifically because of their interest in working with PLWHA. August remembered how his second-year practicum experience inspired a strong desire to search out employment opportunities where he could continue his work with PLWHA. For August, this work was closely connected to the values of the social work profession that appealed to him during his undergraduate studies, particularly the ethical principle of social justice.

Yeah, my internship when I was in the master's program...that's where I really

> got to work with the HIV-positive community and just completely fell in love with that internship and the youth that I was working with. And I really felt comfortable with just the language around HIV care and prevention...And I did not want to leave working within that patient population. I just became very passionate about it, that work. I liked it because I had some friends in my master's program who were in like oncology clinic or in dialysis clinics and it was very medically focused whereas I think in HIV care, there's also a huge social justice component to the work that I was so drawn to. And I think that's true for actually a lot of young clinicians or social workers who get involved in work with the HIV-positive community. I think that there's this social justice piece to it that cannot be ignored when working with folks with HIV. (August)

When August stated that he "did not want to leave working" with PLWHA, he meant it quite literally. His professional trajectory has remained centered on serving this population. Early career experiences can influence the course of a social worker's professional development while simultaneously situating them within the personal, social, and structural forces that define a socioecological approach to practice.

Tony also cited their passion for social justice to explain their interest engaging with PLWHA, while also noting the appeal of working in a medical clinic focused on HIV care. They appreciated that this specialty was better resourced compared to other settings where they worked, including an organization dedicated to the needs of homeless individuals. Tony, who identifies as queer and trans, was also cognizant of how those communities have been disproportionately affected by HIV. They saw their organization as a site where they could pursue their interests with like-minded individuals and serve members of queer communities.

Luca was drawn to their first-year practicum site because they believed it to be a queer-affirming space. They were inspired by an organizational culture that encouraged authenticity among staff and clients.

> And a big factor for me too is working or interning in an organization that had a lot of like openly queer people in it. And yeah, this organization definitely did. I had a really, I felt really comfortable with the person I interviewed with who ended up being my supervisor there. And I felt like I could be myself there, which was a huge, I think, deciding factor in that too. There were some agencies that I interviewed with where they had different standards of professionalism that I don't think, I didn't feel like I would be able to be my authentic queer self there. So, yeah, but I never got that impression with where I ended up. And, yeah, I had a great experience there the entire time. (Luca)

Social work students have faced challenges in their practicums because of homophobic and/or transphobic attitudes and policies, which can lead to distress and discouragement (Messinger et al., 2020). For Luca, placement at this organization was developmentally significant, providing an environment where they could learn how to incorporate their identities with social work knowledge and values and build an affirming approach to social work practice.

Ashley "fell into the HIV space" because of her long-standing interest in working with LGBTQ+ individuals, who she said exist in a "Venn diagram kind of situation" with PLWHA. Similarly, T, when looking for their second-year practicum, knew they wanted to work with LGBTQ+ communities. They estimated that approximately 60% of their PLWHA clients were queer. After many years working in child welfare, Paige observed that her current employment was "the first time in my adult life that I'm working in a queer workplace. And that has been a crazy positive experience for me as a queer person". For these participants, the draw to social work with PLWHA can be explained in part by the close and historical association between HIV and queerness (Argüello, 2023). These accounts suggest that organizations that serve PLWHA offer space where professional commitments and queer identities may converge in ways that make the work personally meaningful.

Other participants had more quotidian reasons for joining their organizations. After graduating with her BSW, Jenny searched for an organization where she could work full-time and would agree to sponsor her advanced practicum.

> Well, I honestly was applying to any jobs after I got my BSW. Also, I needed to find a place where I could do my placement. But my sister previously had worked at, she interned at REDACTED, and she was doing some HIV testing or HIV advocacy work. And so she had spoken to me about this kind of work before. And so, yeah, I kind of like was looking for jobs and I casually found an opening at REDACTED and was like, let's, you know, just give it a try. (Jenny)

Many social work students complete their practicum within their place of employment. These practicums offer many benefits for students who could otherwise not afford to pursue graduate studies, but educators worry about role confusion and the challenges of creating high-quality learning experiences (Lynch et al., 2023).

Simon selected his employer because he qualified for financial assistance to help settle the student loan debt he incurred from his MSW studies.

> Just being totally honest, as an FQHC [Federal Qualified Health Center], there's a

program through HRSA [Health Resources and Services Administration] that provides a loan repayment. And for like X number of years, they give you a lump sum of money towards your loans. That is truly honestly the reason why I applied. (Simon)

Both Jenny and Simon used confessional language ("honest" and "honestly") when explaining what attracted them to their organizations. In both instances, each participant assumed their answers should hearken to loftier ideals about working with PLWHA. By providing "honest" answers, they abandoned pretense. However, their decisions to join these organizations were entirely reasonable. The rationales participants offered span a wide range and reflect considerations rooted in personal preferences, professional development opportunities, and pragmatic need to secure employment.

Job Responsibilities

Participants were asked to share what their work with PLWHA entailed. Medical case management was the most frequently mentioned area of social work with this population. Paige described how she explains medical case management to new clients.

> I'll give you kind of the spiel that I give new clients when I meet with them, like that have never had case management experience. The big picture of my job is to make sure that my clients are attending their appointments as scheduled, and that they are adhering to their medicine, their med regimen and remaining undetectable. So the like big picture, that's what I do. Going down a level, it's, you know, identifying the barriers, the social determinants that are preventing those two main goals from happening and kind of tackling those. Going down another level, it's like identifying needs of my clients and connecting them with resources

that are available to them, whether it's because of their status or regardless of their status. And then, you know, on kind of the basic one-to-one level, it's providing support. (Paige)

While Paige does not explicitly reference ecological theory, her account draws heavily on its core principles. She invoked the language of "levels", echoing the model's structure, and attended to both individual and environmental factors that may facilitate or impede clients' progress, or what she calls "social determinants" (Sprague & Simon, 2021).

Leo, also a medical case manager, described their work as ensuring their clients' HIV is well-maintained and offering general supports and advocacy on behalf of clients.

> I have to keep up with them and their health needs and assess them and do paperwork for the various assessments at different intervals of regularity. And our main goal is treatment adherence, right? And working so I guess like, right, if our main goal is treatment adherence, then the bigger thing is access to their antiretroviral meds, which then is usually benefits stuff. And that's like, I feel like a lot of my role on paper for the reporting that we do to keep my job going. I think it's a lot more than that too, because I think it's being an advocate and a good listener, coming up with ideas and providing referrals. (Leo)

Both Paige and Leo frame medication adherence as a primary responsibility for medical case managers. In Chapter 5, I discuss how social workers navigate adherence. Early career social workers engaged with PLWHA are socialized by their organizations to emphasize the importance of adherence and document their clients' progress with biomedical interventions. Medication adherence extends beyond the interpersonal domain to encompass organizational responsibilities, further demonstrating the need for a socioecological approach to social work with PLWHA.

Several participants offered mental health services to PLWHA. Dan provides behavioral health consulting at a clinic dedicated to the needs of PLWHA. He described his role as a collaborator with medical providers to address the mental health needs of clients in the clinical setting.

> So I do behavioral health consulting. So I'm doing brief interventions with kids, adults, and families. We also work with babies. And so sometimes, you know, and we're basically just trying to offer screeners depending on screener results, referrals, and then we also do targeted kind of more short-term interventions. We do offer bridge therapy as well. So, if we connect someone to a clinic, we could hypothetically offer therapy for like a few sessions in the interim. But it's more set up as brief supports for people. (Dan)

Josh offered psychotherapy at a community mental health center. Josh currently works with two PLWHA clients, following his assignment to several queer-identified clients.

> They had a huge waitlist when I showed up and they just ran these like, find all the gay and trans clients and gave them to me, showed up, and they're like, oh, you've also experienced doing it. Yeah, and then, because I have a history of working in drug and alcohol, they gave me a bunch of drug and alcohol clients. And kind of since then, I just really dived headfirst into doing, getting trained in and doing more trauma-focused therapy. So that is a big focus of my work now is like EMDR and somatic experiencing and just like trauma specific trauma focused therapy work. (Josh)

Josh described being pigeonholed as an expert on LGBTQ+ populations, which can be both an opportunity and burden (Nelson et al., 2026). As an early career social worker entering their first professional social work job post-graduation, it is possible Josh felt more pressure to accept certain clients. As Josh gained more experience and confidence, they participated in trauma-focused trainings to build a knowledge base applicable across client populations, rather than limiting their work to specific groups.

Scott formerly worked in homeless services. His program did not specialize in HIV services, but he estimated he worked with between 50 and 100 PLWHA during his time there. Scott described an array of services and interventions he offered to clients while he was engaged with this program.

> And it was an overnight emergency shelter program. And I was the case manager for the program. And so I was responsible for doing intakes and housing-focused case management and helping acquire documentation. In broad terms, that was what the role consisted of, intakes, engagement, housing-focused case management, documentation, some community management in terms of spending time in the shelter and engaging people, and some outreach with different programs to build a relationship with the shelter and engage with people who were living on the street and who may be interested in coming into shelter but hesitant until they speak with someone who can describe the shelter firsthand. (Scott)

Participants' stories highlight that social work with PLWHA is multifaceted, spanning diverse settings, interventions, and responsibilities in response to the complex needs of varied client populations.

Job Satisfaction

Job satisfaction compromises the cognitive, affective, and behavioral components an individual draws upon to evaluate their overall attitude about their employment, which can range from positive to negative (Judge et al., 2020; Pugh, 2016). Participants were asked about their satisfaction with their work and organizations. Generally, participants noted how much they enjoyed their work and appreciated their employers. Ashley, whose entire social work career has focused on the needs of PLWHA, stated that her familiarity with the HIV social work infrastructure, along with her passion for the work, has sustained her within medical case management settings.

> This is gonna sound weird, but it's really fun. Like, I think HIV doctors are inherently cool. Like they're cooler than like, like if you wanna be an HIV doctor, like that's, that tells me that you're like, at least somewhat socially conscious. It's, it's a space that I've felt comfortable in. I also kind of nailed down the terminology and the lingo, like viral load and CD4 and all this kind of stuff and opportunistic infection and whatever. And also the resources, I know this food pantry, I know this program, I know what Ryan White covers, like it's just, and I love medical social work. So it's all just kind of, it makes sense. It made sense to me to stay with that. (Ashley)

As Ashley became more acclimated to the demands of her role, she gained confidence, contributing to a sense of job satisfaction that has sustained her work with PLWHA across different organizations and settings.

Winnie, who also works in medical case management, shared how they found meaning in their work, which was a pleasant change from previous corporate roles that left them deeply unsatisfied.

> I feel fulfilled by what I'm doing, and that has been what I like have been looking for in a job, in a career...There are some days when I do feel like overwhelmed, burntout, like oh my God, but then I come home and I cuddle with [my dog] and then it's all okay. But like overall I just really stick to that fulfilled feeling because that again has just like been what I have been searching for since college when I joined the corporate marketing field and just hated that. This is so different, and I love it. (Winnie)

Winnie discovered a sense of purpose in their work that validated their decision to pursue social work. For early career social workers, such moments may serve as important affirmations of their emerging professional identity.

Dan's work in an HIV clinic is a radical professional departure. He found himself rejuvenated working in a compassionate environment with dedicated colleagues.

> I would say this place for me was a, I don't know if reprieve, but it was recovery from almost all the other settings I've been in…Like, this is like a place I actually look forward to working in. It's a place that I enjoy coming to work to be around coworkers who I'm really close with. And I think even how the treatment of patients, I think, reflects that too, where there is a respect, where there is a kindness that is shown that feels very different than, especially because I've worked in more substance use spaces as well, there's still somewhat of like this punitive old school vibe at times. So, yeah, it just feels like night and day at times. (Dan)

A high level of organizational commitment is associated with less burnout and less likelihood of turnover (Brown et al., 2019). Ashley, Winnie, and Dan's allegiance to their employers highlights how workplace settings that offer personal and professional benefits can foster commitment. Given enduring retention challenges (Alboroto et al., 2025; Pulman & Fenge, 2025), such environments may play a pivotal role in influencing early career social workers' professional development and career trajectories.

Other participants noted the association between work-life balance and job satisfaction. Simon has been with his current employer for many years. When asked why he stays, he noted his position is not overly demanding of his time and mental resources.

> What has made me stay is the quality of life, the work-life balance. By no means am I stressed at work. It's pretty straightforward. It's great benefits. I'm not stressed. Yeah, I would say it's really the work-life balance that it provides. (Simon)

But for Lynn, who has only been with their employer for less than six months, establishing work-life balance has been difficult. They worry that their position may not be sustainable long-term. Lynn's economic anxieties negatively impact their job satisfaction.

> There are parts that aren't the most fun, but I think that's in any job...I do like it, again, the pay isn't great...I would hope, I was told that it doesn't really increase as well, so that's something that might be an issue for me, you know, maybe after a year, unfortunately. I would hope it wouldn't, but you know, I also have to take care of myself and pay my bills and save hopefully, you know, all the things that we all need to do. So that's kind of my only larger issue with it is just if I can stay here long-term because of that. I also work other jobs. So I feel like I have to figure out that balance just if I can stay here long-term because of that. How many

other jobs can I work with doing this and finding that balance? (Lynn)

Early career social workers often enter the profession with lofty ideals, but find themselves saddled with debt and low salaries (Apgar & Dolan, 2023). Job satisfaction is not a substitute for equitable compensation.

August recalled his disappointment with his first post-MSW position working with PLWHA. While he enjoyed working with clients, inadequate wages, untenable workplace conditions, and emotional exhaustion caused significant turnover in staff.

> It was very rewarding. It also paid terribly…it just feels so criminal to me that we got paid that little to work that hard. Because of the amount of paperwork that we were doing, it was tons of paperwork, so there would be days where I would have to stay until 10 p.m. at night to catch up on all of my notes and making sure I was having all the files I needed. Because I wasn't just a care coordinator there, I was also the lead clinician and also a therapist and also worked for their outpatient clinic in addition to their day program. So I had many hats there. So what I think was hard about, the work was hard, yes, because it was so complex. And the clients had so many complex issues in addition to their health, just like family dynamics, relational dynamics, very significant mental health issues, and then the challenges of working in a very low-funded mental health center. Yeah, there's a ton of turnover in that staff there. (August)

Salaries for social workers remain low compared to their colleagues in other helping professions (Hughes et al., 2018; Lewis, 2018); Wilfong (2024) argues low pay for social workers is a human rights violation. Insufficient salaries, in conjunction with job stress and burnout, are predictive of turnover (Abu- Bader, 2000). The profession's history of low pay and low status, gendered in nature, combined with educational practices (such as unpaid practicums) that disadvantage students, may force social workers to seek more sustainable employment (Hodge et al., 2024).

Nora acknowledged she is struggling in her current position and shared that the cumulative affective nature of the work impacts her ability to perform. She remembered a recent incident working with a client with a long history of substance use. Her client was disrespectful and dismissive of Nora's offers of assistance.

> I cannot see myself doing it much longer. It's emotionally taxing and I'm getting to a point where I'm afraid that I'm not being effective. Like this client I was just talking about who relapsed, like that my personal frustrations are getting in the way of me being a good case manager, and I don't want that. Yeah, I don't know how much longer I can stay in it. (Nora)

While she did not use the word, Nora's current state might be described as burnout, defined as a state of emotional exhaustion, negative feelings about clients, and a decreased sense of occupational efficacy (Frieiro Padín et al., 2021; Maddock, 2024). Higher levels of burnout are associated with lower levels of job satisfaction (Gómez-García et al., 2021; Zhang & He, 2022). The challenges inherent in social work with PLWHA, including psychosocial stressors and organizational constraints, contribute to burnout (Jones et al., 2022; Reid et al., 2024). Organizations looking to retain a competent and caring workforce must consider the importance of job satisfaction. While all social workers could use more organizational support, this is more critical for early career social workers who may feel overwhelmed and unprepared for their new responsibilities (Hochman et al., 2023).

Supervision

Participants reflected upon their experiences on the job (as opposed to practicum) receiving supervision. Social work supervision is broadly conceptualized as a working relationship between a supervisor and supervisee designed to develop the supervisee's social work competence through the use of educational, administrative, and supportive practices (Kaplan et al., 2025). Participants had decidedly mixed experiences with supervision. Some participants valued the advice and instruction they received, while others shared that they had little or no supervision, or supervision that did not meet their needs. Jenny recalled a recent incident with a client who claimed she was not working hard enough to find them housing. She internalized this criticism and found herself becoming emotional. Jenny shared how her supervisor worked with her and the client to resolve the matter.

> And so my supervisor really helped him understand or helped us understand where the client was coming from and really laid out the groundwork for the client to have clear expectations of what I as a medical case manager can do and some of the things that were expected of him. But yeah, that was like a core memory in my social work career that I will always remember. And my supervisor was super helpful to me. Then we later on debriefed after the client was no longer here and she helped me really understand how like situations like that can sometimes happen when clients may not have a clear understanding of what the case manager can do for them or sometimes they're just feeling frustrated of so many things that are happening in their life that they may have these emotions and how we can help them navigate for them not to feel that way anymore. (Jenny)

Jenny's supervisor provided educational and supportive interventions that allowed Jenny and her client to better understand the role of the medical case manager. In describing this moment as a "core memory in my social work career that I will always remember", Jenny illustrated how positive, encouraging supervision can build competence and confidence, thereby enhancing professional development.

Paige stressed that having a good supervisor was very important in her role as a medical case manager.

> But I also cannot overstate the importance of having a good supervisor, which I know is kind of beyond the control of many social workers, but I have a wonderful supervisor who is truly a mentor. And, you know, like I've had shitty supervisors, of course. A lot of supervisors are people that got like shoved into their role because they've been around the longest. But I have a really wonderful supervisor, and her supervisor is excellent, is one of us, our department director, you know. So when I have challenging moments at work, the first thing I do is I talk to the supervisors around and they have supported me in my role. But also my colleagues are close friends, personally, so having good colleagues really helps as well. (Paige)

Paige's close relationships with her supervisor and colleagues offer her the support necessary to address the more difficult aspects of her work. Such support is a developmental resource that builds confidence and defines her professional identity over time.

Emma was displeased with a supervisor more concerned about meeting client targets than offering encouragement. She referred to the grief she experienced when clients died and the lack of an empathetic response from her supervisor.

> I don't feel like my supervision currently addresses it very well. I think in the past it has at my job, but, and they've tried to like launch like monthly counseling and grief groups for people who work as case managers…but it didn't like kind of take off. I think just like not enough people made it a priority to show up every month. And so it wasn't maintained, but I think there could be more support for that, especially on my team specifically, because we just deal with a lot of that, just the nature of the population that we work with…I work with difficult clients and it's like a lot and there's burnout and compassion fatigue. I would like more emotional support and less focus on numbers and data and stuff like that. (Emma)

Emma desired supervision that was fully attentive to her needs and the challenges inherent in medical case management. In addition to burnout, Emma used the term "compassion fatigue", defined as negative consequences of working with traumatized clients, including reduced capacity for empathy and presence with clients (Adams et al., 2006; Harr et al., 2014). While the two terms are often used interchangeably, burnout is a reaction in response to organizational stressors, while compassion fatigue involves the vicarious effects that may arise from exposure to clients' traumas (Thomas, 2013). Emma's response suggests that effective supervision, attuned to affective needs, is lacking at her organization. Early career social workers require positive reinforcement and support from supervisors as an essential part of their professional growth (Apgar & Dolan, 2023).

Participants stressed that what they most valued in supervision was the personal contact between supervisor and social worker. The findings suggest that participants favored relational engagement over technical guidance or administrative oversight. Nora stated that supervision "was a place to vent", where she could seek counsel to address "annoying" situations and learn how to manage her feelings. Similarly, Paige felt that her supervision was a balance of administrative tasks and emotional support, but leaned more heavily into the latter.

> I would, I mean, I would say a mix of the two. Like really, I just go in, I kind of talk about what I've got going on. I keep my supervisor updated on situations that are unfolding with my clients. She will ask me questions that I haven't thought about or have you asked them this, think about it this way, try this. She just gives me feedback and then she will ask me, she'll be checking in on clients I haven't heard from in a while, stuff like that. I guess I would say 70-30 emotional support and feedback. (Paige)

For other participants, supervision was miserable. August clearly recalled his negative experiences with a supervisor at his first post-MSW job in community mental health. He shared his supervisor mistreated him in several ways, making his time at a stressful workplace even more difficult.

> Yeah, I dreaded supervision…I mean, it felt like I was being grilled. I felt like I had to learn a lot because I felt like when I was going into supervision, if I didn't know something about HIV, if there was something about HIV, whether it was biomedical, whether it was like literally anything, shame on me for not knowing. So I had to do a ton of learning out of fear. So I would never treat staff that way. I think that's why I'm like, no, you need to, you're going to learn, but you need to be very humble in the work. (August)

August understood at an early stage of his professional development what kind of supervisor he wanted to be. In drawing upon humility as his touchstone, August celebrated curiosity and learning as important elements of supervision, as opposed to an inflexible and unhelpful expectation of perfectionism that he experienced at the outset of his social work career.

Intra-Organization Collaboration

Most participants worked at medium-sized to large organizations where their work often depended on close partnerships with colleagues. Participants were asked to offer examples of working together with other professionals within their organizations. Collaboration, a cooperative enterprise where multiple professionals achieve outcomes beyond those that could be delivered by individuals alone, is an important element of social work that should be introduced in MSW classroom and practicum education (Bronstein, 2003; D'Agostino, 2013; Milano et al., 2022). Most examples of collaboration were offered by participants employed in medical case management. Most participants stated that they had good working relationships with medical providers within their organizations, but role confusion and different professional philosophies presented challenges. Nora shared frustration over the ignorance of providers as to the psychosocial stressors clients experience.

> I think what I'm noticing lately is that we get a lot of the social service things that are going on with the client, whereas the provider gets obviously all of the medical, very much the science of it. So a provider might say, please go see GI, urology, etc., etc., and we'll try to do that on our end, but on our end, that looks like making the appointment. Client doesn't go. Scheduling another one. Client

> doesn't go. Us trying to address those barriers, client not answering the phone, us not being able to reach a client. So there is still a lot of disconnect just because our roles are different and we have a perspective that the providers don't and maybe the providers have a perspective that we don't. (Nora)

Nora was grateful that her organization has internal systems that allowed for efficient communication between social workers and medical providers; she praised the accessibility of the medical providers with whom she works. Differences in status, priorities, and socialization can hinder collaboration between social workers and physicians, although both groups can effectively work together (Abramson & Mizrahi, 2003).

Paige believed that her clients were often uncertain about the different responsibilities of social workers and medical providers, a confusion that can impact expectations of care and require social workers to continually clarify their role in interdisciplinary settings. She stated that providers and social workers need to function as a team to ensure optimal client outcomes.

> In my experience, you know, I mean, we have such different roles. Like, I'm not a doctor. Sometimes my clients will ask me, like, medical questions, and I'm like, girl, what? Like, ask your doctor. I don't know. And same thing with the providers. Like, I've been in visits where a chronically homeless client will look at their doctor and say, can you help me? I need an ID. And I'll be like, why are you at, like, he doesn't know how to do that. Let me know. And for the most part, like, there's definitely a mutual understanding and respect there of like, this is what you do. And I need you. It's a very, like, kind of symbiotic relationship. We need each other and we rely on each other to do our jobs. The providers definitely rely on us

to make their jobs easier. (Paige)

Participants stated that their collaboration with medical providers was often impeded by poor communication. Winnie recalled how one of the social workers they supervised discovered that a client was deceased.

> One of my case managers recently had a situation where he found out one of his clients, who was both a case management client and a health center client, he found out that she was deceased because he went into her health center portal and it said deceased, when the provider should have called the case manager when learning that and submitted an incident report. And there's all these policies and all these things that should have happened. And if that had happened on our end, we would have done all that and let the provider know. So that was really frustrating and really unfair to the case manager. (Winnie)

Nora recalled a similar experience. She noted that doctors are often the first to learn about a client's death and the social worker is the last to know. At her organization, providers "turn off" a client's electronic file when they learn of their passing; no notice is sent to the social worker. Nora felt that, although this practice has become "normalized", her organization could do better. Death notification is a sensitive matter that can have repercussions for both the recipient and reporter (De Leo et al., 2023). Social workers may experience a range of emotions upon learning of the death of a client, including self- blame, anger, shock, and helplessness (Hung et al., 2023); social workers at the beginning of their career may be especially vulnerable. The stories of Winnie and Nora suggest that organizations need to pay more attention to their policies and procedures around death notification, not only to ensure ethical and compassionate practice but also to support the professional development of social workers negotiating grief, communication, and role expectations during challenging moments.

Participants also discussed their collaboration with their fellow social workers and the close-knit bonds that develop on their teams. Overall, participants reported positive working relationships with colleagues. Leo talked about how they and their colleagues work together to handle client situations when the assigned social worker may be out of the office.

> Like, if you know someone's out and maybe this [client] isn't on my caseload, but I know their situation more than the rest of the team because I like am kind of their-ish, you know, so that's kind of when I'll step in and help and vice versa, you know, like we kind of, it's just kind of whoever meets that guy next or something, but yeah, we all work very closely together. (Leo)

When Leo stated that they might be another client's "ish", they meant that they may have a pre-existing relationship or some knowledge of the client and their particular situation. Leo remembered sharing with their colleagues their system for tracking their caseload which was them adopted throughout the organization, illustrating how early career social workers can contribute to organizational practice through innovation and exchange with peers.

Lynn desired more collaboration at their organization. They suggested that early career social workers could benefit from mentorship programs that are more supportive and peer-driven and less connected to client outcomes and organizational mandates. They missed the relationships they had created during their MSW program and sought a suitable replacement.

> I just think as a new social worker and in any field and especially in, you know, medical case management, HIV care, I think it would be really helpful to have like mentorships. I think that's something that I have always kind of been looking for and haven't really been able to have maybe through lack of my own advocacy, maybe through just not sure how to navigate that...But yeah, it would be nice to have more community as new social workers. I think sometimes you're at a school and maybe you don't have those connections from school anymore, maybe you do. It would just be nice to have that support of learning and growing together. (Lynn)

The transition from student to professional social worker can be a time of stress and confusion for even the most prepared individual (Cleveland et al., 2019). Lynn appreciated the trainings they received as a new employee but recognized they missed the supports they received while in school. Social work mentorship programs can promote wellbeing and resilience in early career social workers and offer opportunities to address concerns such as burnout or low job satisfaction (Boddy et al., 2012; Popowa, 2024; Toh et al., 2018). Given the stressors that come with medical case management with PLWHA, Lynn's suggestion for mentorship is worth further exploration.

Ramifications of HIV Diagnosis

In her research into the lives of women living with HIV, Watkins-Hayes (2019) explores how HIV inspired transformative projects; or, as one individual memorably put it, "if it weren't for HIV, I'd probably be dead" (p. 1). After learning their diagnosis, these women were caught by an HIV safety net consisting of services and resources woven together to promote the health and dignity of PLWHA. However, access to this safety net requires a diagnosis previously understood as a harbinger of death. Several participants noted the seeming incongruity that a person needed to contract a potentially fatal virus to access life-affirming supports.

> And I think the place I work, I think it's interesting, I think HIV work is sometimes more resourced than other settings, especially from coming with, from working with folks who are unhoused. So like there is a lot more funding and like research and like attention in some ways. (Tony)

Given recent efforts to eliminate or severely cut funding for PLWHA, it is unknown whether systems of care will be able to provide the same level of resources that have sustained this community for decades.

Scott, in his work with homeless individuals, recognized that PLWHA were prioritized in programs designed to address housing insecurity.

> What was particularly strange in the homeless services system, to some extent, a person having a diagnosis of HIV was beneficial in terms of being able to access certain streams of housing support that others would not access. And it generally seemed like people who had a diagnosis of HIV could get access to housing more quickly. So in some ways, when a person would come in and we would do an intake and talk with them and they would reveal, oh, by the way, I also have HIV, in some ways I would think, oh, this could actually be good for you for resolving your housing crisis because it demonstrates you are more of a priority. You are a special population that the city and or federal government recognizes, deserves to be prioritized. And so it was odd to sometimes be in a position of saying, yes, having HIV is a chronic health condition you have to live with and manage, but in terms of your housing crisis, this could be a good card to have. (Scott)

Stable housing has long been known to be an important intervention to improve the lives of PLWHA and prevent new infections (Aidala & Sumartojo, 2007; Stone et al., 2022). Scott also acknowledged that for most of his PLWHA homeless clients, HIV was not a major issue of concern and their viral loads and CD4 counts were well managed. Programs and organizations dedicated to the needs of PLWHA trace their histories back to the worst days of the HIV epidemic (Schulman, 2021). Scott recognized some dissonance, using words such as "strange" and "odd", to describe this situation. He previously shared that when he was growing up, HIV was considered "the biggest and the baddest", but that was not how his PLWHA clients experienced the virus. Scott understood HIV not as a fatal illness, but a manageable condition that served as a gateway to housing. Specialized programs designed to meet certain needs and populations are not unusual, but as ideas and opinions about HIV change, the fate of these programs may be increasingly called into question. In Chapter 8, I explore the question of whether HIV is still considered an exceptional condition.

An HIV diagnosis also provides access to safe and affirmative spaces. Dan shared that many clients at his clinic have received services there for many years, and in some cases, since birth. He described his organization as a sanctuary, a place where individuals could receive compassionate care in a familiar and comfortable community setting.

> So it's weird, this is kind of a mixed thing, and I want to be careful how I like articulate this, but I think there's ways in which, in the context of our clinic becoming involved, that HIV has almost created a lifeline to supports and opportunities that patients wouldn't have otherwise had. So, I'm by no means trying to, like, romanticize, but I do think our clinic is a really impressive,

> thoughtful space. As someone working there, I've really enjoyed the experience, but also the patients who come in, they feel like this is part of their family, and not in like a totally dysfunctional toxic way, but it's a really, it's like a really remarkable space. And so I do think it's unfortunate that this is their entry point to getting connections and support. (Dan)

His description of the organization as "part of their family" suggests the depth of the connections that clients, social workers, and other helpers create within this space, revealing how systems of care can become sites of belonging fashioned by relationship and shared experiences.

Billy revealed that, when he was working at a recovery home, he had clients tell him that they wanted to be infected with HIV to access benefits and services. While there are individuals who have deliberately sought out HIV (Grov & Parsons, 2006; Moskowitz & Roloff, 2007; Tewksbury, 2006), there are few known cases involving individuals who expressed a financial motive. Billy noted these individuals were younger and less knowledgeable about HIV.

> Well, the younger generation, I mean, I think they realize that having HIV gives them access to benefits that a lot of other people don't have. And I actually had two individuals who wanted to get HIV because it made housing available, it gave them the ability to be on a list to get housing, gave them benefits that other people don't have. (Billy)

Billy, an HIV activist with deep connections to PLWHA communities, was asked what it felt like for him to hear clients express a wish to become infected.

> It feels two different ways, right? So I'm happy for them that they have the

> benefits and also, they have the benefits because I got my ass arrested. Because I died in the street. Because of the work I and other people did in ACT UP. You know? And that's great, you know, and I'm grateful for that. But it also, I don't, I've never been angry about it, but I've also just been like, wow, you know, like I lost so many people who didn't get the benefits that they are getting. And getting those benefits comes from a very entitled place and that doesn't always feel good. (Billy)

Billy recognized that many younger individuals have no appreciation for the history of the epidemic and the possible consequences of HIV. Even with medical advancements, HIV remains a serious health challenge not to be taken lightly (Allan-Blitz et al., 2021; Fernandez et al., 2021). Billy's perspective, informed by years of personal experience with PLWHA, was more conflicted than that of other participants who had not witnessed the damage caused by the virus, suggesting that exposure to the epidemic's earlier devastation shapes meaning making and professional orientation over time.

Role of the Organization for Clients

Participants stated their thoughts about the role their organizations play in the lives of PLWHA clients. Overall, they believed clients had developed strong bonds with organizations that play a significant role in their lives. Nora remarked that her organization has provided support for PLWHA for decades. For her clients, the organization was a place of stability during chaotic times.

> I mean, for some clients, we have been a constant. And, you know, as it happens anywhere, there are people who come and they sort of get comfortable, and we get to know their names and they know our names, and so they feel seen. So yeah, I

think we've played an important role for people. I just met someone today who gets tested for HIV periodically. He came in nine months ago or got tested nine months ago somewhere else. He was negative, came in last week on Friday, and he was positive for HIV. And he said, I just Googled, I just found you guys on Google for free testing and I came in. And so…the fact that he was able to find us, come in, do the test and we were able to talk to him right away, like I think that's valuable. So for our long-term clients and also new clients, I think we provide value in that way, that we are here. (Nora)

Nora stressed that, even with a decline in HIV incidence, there is a substantial number of individuals who rely on organizations like hers to provide life-sustaining services for older PLWHA and linkages to care for newly diagnosed individuals. Even with the changes in the epidemic, organizations that serve PLWHA have continuing value.

Derek recalled his second-year placement where he facilitated a specialized program designed to meet the mental health needs of PLWHA. He noted the isolation and loneliness that many PLWHA experience and how this unique location offered community, connections, and safety.

I have people that have been living with [HIV] for, you know, over a decade and nobody knew. Their family didn't know. Someone had a spouse and their spouse didn't know. So it was this intensely secret part of themselves, and this was the only space where they could identify openly in that way and find communities, community with others. You know, so important. A lot of these folks lived alone and were unemployed so just community in general was really hard for them and this is where they would go to find that. And you know, a lot of them were friends…so it was really this idea of the third space or whatever, it was really that for them. So community around HIV/AIDS, yes, but also just community in general, you know. This is really special in that regard. (Derek)

Derek may be drawing upon the work of Oldenburg (2001), who described the "third space" as a location beyond home and the workplace where individuals gather freely and frequently. Oldenburg argues that these spaces—low cost, accessible, and leveling (status differences are minimized)—are fundamental to improve health and foster community. While not using the same terminology, Dan emphasized the supportive and special nature of the clinic where he works.

> So it's a weird thing, because in many ways, it [becoming HIV-positive] obviously is an entirely life-altering experience. But I think in a lot of cases, it has been the result of a life that was lived in somewhat of an isolated, secretive space where folks were engaging in ways without maybe as much of an awareness of how to sometimes safely practice sex. And so, I do think when they enter a clinic, it is initially traumatizing. It's a huge, huge thing, obviously, for most of our patients. But I've worked with a lot of folks for whom this is part of their home, part of their family. So, it has offered an opportunity for support. And I don't know, almost like an opportunity for them to also come into their own in a way that I don't know how they would have outside of that. It's just such a unique space. (Dan)

Secrecy, especially in the context of HIV, can have a negative impact on health and wellbeing, as well as serve as a protective factor (Fielden et al., 2011; Galano et al., 2017). For Derek and Dan, their organizations were places where individuals could live more authentic lives without fear of judgment or reprisal. Similarly, Simon saw his organization as a refuge where clients knew "I'm not going to be turned away. I'm not going to be looked at differently because I have HIV". In a world where discrimination based on HIV status is still prevalent (Feyissa et al., 2019; Karver et al., 2022; Logie et al., 2018), organizations that serve PLWHA are vitally needed.

Other participants noted that their organizations offer a unique "one-stop" model where clients can have multiple needs addressed in a single visit. Leo shared how one client's medical appointment could set off a chain reaction of social worker contacts and resources.

> Yeah, they can receive their medical care there, or they could just receive their case management services there with me and go to the doctor somewhere else. They could also get their prescriptions at our pharmacy, or they could go somewhere else too, but we like to give them options. A lot of people do like to one-stop shop it, and it's fun. Like someone will show up for a doctor's appointment, leave having had a coffee with their case manager and an entire bag of food from the food pantry. Maybe I stole them a sweater, you know, or something somewhere, and they'll have, you know, will only pick and choose one service or two. (Leo)

Observing caring, efficient, client-centered social work in these settings early in their professional lives may help early career social workers develop a broader understanding of how medical, material, and personal supports intersect in clients' lives, reinforcing a socioecological perspective on practice. They may also come to see that clients are often connected not only to individual providers, but to the organization itself as a place of safety and continuity.

Organizational Responses to Current Events

The second Trump Administration has resulted in momentous changes in policy, strategy, and tone that stand in stark contrast to its predecessors. In Chapter 8, I address how the administration's policies impact PLWHA and the organizations that serve them. Participants were asked how their organizations responded to shifting priorities and financial threats emanating from Washington D.C. Participants were generally unsatisfied but suggested that anxiety and a lack of clarity complicated these efforts. Emma shared that her organization, which relies heavily on federal funding, has not offered clear messaging about current events.

> You know, they haven't mentioned it much. Like, they've, I've had clients ask about it, and I just am transparent with them that I know as much as they do probably. And they just like, haven't really shared many kind of predictions for the future. They're just kind of like, we don't know, we're taking it day by day. Which is also, you know, it's a lot of uncertainty, I think. (Emma)

Simon said that his organization was still trying to find its footing after the COVID-19 pandemic. The combination of challenges from both within and outside of the organization hampered a definitive, coordinated response.

> COVID hit us hard financially, and, you know, certain financial moves that perhaps should have happened didn't happen. We're currently under new leadership. So while we try to adjust internally, we're now also facing the external stressors. So, conversations have been had, and when changes are going to come, what they are right now, it's hard to say because of, we got some internal stuff to figure out, but now that's complicated because we don't know what's happening

externally and how that's going to impact dollars. (Simon)

Participants see that recent actions and rhetoric have affected their organizations. Winnie shared how they and their colleagues are supporting each other during difficult moments.

> There's definitely been kind of a constant air of just stress, uncertainty, some just burnout amongst my colleagues, which is normal in this field anyway, but I think exacerbated by all the uncertainty, governmentally and just worldwide. So yeah, it can definitely be tough, but there is a really, really good like community among the staff and people are really like looking out for each other. So I think that helps to mitigate all the stress that people are holding. (Winnie)

Winnie emphasized that they and their colleagues focus on what is within their control and allow their supervisors and other administrators to address other matters. The orientation toward mutual support reflects how early career social workers learn how to address uncertainty in a collective manner.

Other participants remarked that their organizations were communicating with as much candor as possible. Tony stated that they appreciated how their organization was responding in the moment, even with limited information and guidance available.

> I think we talk about it pretty openly. Fortunately, our directors are pretty transparent and will say, you know, like, this is what the funders are telling us and this is where we're at. And I think we have been kind of talking about, like, what we can do to look for, for like other funding to try to bill insurance more if possible and sustain our work in the ways we can. (Tony)

This openness, even in the absence of certainty, demonstrates how transparency functions as an organizational resource and intervention, assisting early career social workers to make sense of changing conditions and maintain a commitment to client care.

Leo was unhappy with their organization's response to current events. They work for a medium-sized organization well-known in their community for their work with PLWHA. Leo believed their organization pre-emptively capitulated to the new administration.

> Yeah, so, they scrubbed the website. The mission statement, the words Black and Brown, I think HIV, I think it just says we do social services and case management and healthcare. Doesn't say gender affirming care, doesn't even say LGBT, like they got rid of everything. It's big as hell and yeah, I think they folded pretty fast in my opinion...I don't know what I would do if I was in that position of having to make decisions and being worried about a loss of funding if your website says the wrong words…But at the same time if we fold, what does that say to our clients, you know what I mean? I think about like that from like a trauma-informed lens too and I'm like, come on guys. I don't know but yeah there was definitely a discussion but honestly there was only one discussion. They were like this is what's happening and we're gonna pretend to tell you what's going on, but like, we're not really going to tell you the details, you know, that was kind of how it was handled. (Leo)

Leo believed the organization failed to uphold its values and history and acted contrary to the best interests of clients. By specifically noting that the organization's approach was not aligned with trauma-informed principles (Bent-Goodley, 2019; Knight, 2015; Levenson, 2017), Leo drew upon their social work background to contextualize their organization's approach. At the time of the interviews for this project, the second

Trump Administration was in its first few months. Further research is necessary to understand how ASOs are surviving (or not) as the political arena becomes even more contentious.

Conclusion

Organizations shape how care is delivered to PLWHA, how social workers are supported, and how institutional values are put into practice. Attending to the organizational level of the socioecological model focuses on how workplace structures, policies, and cultures impact client outcomes and social worker wellbeing. Social workers who assume a socioecological approach may be better positioned to advocate for clients, pursue systematic change, and develop professionally over time.

Chapter 7
Community-Level HIV Contexts

Within the socioecological model, community-level factors capture the social norms, personal and professional relationships, and institutional contexts that affect social work experiences beyond the individual or organization. For social workers engaged with PLWHA, stigma emerges as a particularly significant phenomenon that impacts how clients access resources and reinforces health and social inequities. Social workers engaged with PLWHA tend to stigmas directed at race, sexual orientation, gender identity, and other forms of marginalization. An examination of stigma from acommunity-level perspective provides early career social workers with important lessons about how barriers to care and wellbeing are socially organized, rather than the result of the perceived failings of clients. This chapter focuses on two themes centered on community-level factors: collaboration with outside providers; and stigma emanating from local communities.

Collaboration with Outside Providers

When participants needed to work with partner organizations, medical providers, or governmental agencies in their communities on behalf of clients, their efforts were hampered by poor communication. Integrated cross-system collaborations are considered essential for improved client outcomes, but alliances can be derailed by role confusion, clashes between organizational cultures, differing priorities and practices, and underdeveloped facilitation of successful partnerships (Bunger et al., 2024; Fleming et al., 2023; Van Eck et al., 2024; van Muijden et al., 2025). Lynn was frustrated with healthcare providers who failed to timely respond to requests for necessary documentation or medication refills.

> I have a little difficulty sometimes reaching people. Mainly my collaboration is, if someone is telling me they aren't able to get a refill or something, and they're asking me to advocate a little, I keep calling, I'm not getting on, can you call? Like, yeah, sure, I don't mind stepping in sometimes and if they ask around that, if they're like really frustrated, they can't get in contact with someone. Or just for labs, to be in our program, we have to have labs at least once a year. We really do it like twice and be connected to medical care like once or twice a year…So yeah, I would say 99%, great. But there's that 1% where sometimes you're like, oh, I just can't get through to anyone. I've been calling and I've sent five different faxes. And at that time, sometimes I need the client to advocate a little bit for themselves to be like, hey, can you just call and let them know and that we really need this for this program. And then for the most time, then that it works when they call and request it to be sent. (Lynn)

Lynn understood that clients may need to intercede when organizational barriers limit the social worker's ability to meet client needs, illustrating how access to care is often relies upon both professional advocacy and clients' own capacity to maneuver complex healthcare systems. Clients' self-advocacy efforts are addressed in Chapter 5.

Participants noted that collaboration with outside providers was often time-intensive and frustrating. Winnie recalled when one of their supervisees had a difficult time verifying a client's HIV diagnosis. They discovered they could not always rely upon outside providers to address basic requests in a reasonable time frame.

> Definitely challenging when it's an external health center. I know a lot of times, case managers have reached out to try to get lab work, or they have to get a confirmation of the HIV diagnosis when clients are doing their intake in order to get them Ryan White certified in order to participate in case management. And I know one of my case managers recently got a referral, and she's reached out to the provider five times to try to get this confirmation of diagnosis, and they keep sending everything but that. So sometimes they're not helpful at all. Sometimes providers are the worst. (Winnie)

For early career social workers, one of the most challenging tasks in their professional development is navigating complex systems and inter-organization collaborations while concurrently adapting to new responsibilities and identities (Davidson & Darracott, 2024). Leo came to understand they are often powerless to compel others to perform their duties.

> I mean, it's a little frustrating. But it's also like there is a small sense of, well, it's out of my hands. I did my bit, you know. But it's definitely like you have to also hear and empathize with the client and you know hopelessness is hard to not kind of pick up too, but at the same time it's like, yeah I know these are the systems. To know at least I'm not the one doing the gatekeeping is, well, okay. (Leo)

Leo recognized that continued delay on the part of outside organizations requires helping clients not get stuck in a maddening morass of sluggish systems. Recognizing that they are not the cause of the problem ("I know these are the systems") allows Leo to focus on what is within their control. This distinction anchors Leo to what is actionable within their immediate spheres of influence, even when larger systems are unhelpful. The experiences of participants suggest that education and support around inter-organizational collaboration should be incorporated into student classroom and practicum learning (Barr et al., 2024).

Stigma

Social workers require knowledge of the substantial impact of stigma in the lives of PLWHA. Stigma is a multilayered, multidimensional construct that enforces social inequality by means of discrimination, stereotyping, and labeling of individuals and groups based upon some perceived negative trait or characteristic (Earnshaw et al., 2013; Edelman et al., 2017; Johnson Shen et al., 2019). While Goffman (1963) refers to stigma as "an attribute that is deeply discrediting", he emphasizes that "a language of relationships, not attributes, is really needed" (p. 3). Goffman argues the meaning of stigma is not fixed in stone, but contingent upon the setting where and when an encounter takes place; stigma is better understood to be a *relationship* between an attribute and a stereotype.

Link and Phelan (2001) assert that most studies of stigma are too centered on individual-level processes. They propose a definition of stigma composed of five components: labeling of human differences; connection of difference to a negative stereotype; separation of those with the stigma from those without; experiences of discrimination and loss of status; and the exercise of social, economic, and political power against the stigmatized. Link and colleagues (2004) add emotional reactions, such as feelings of embarrassment, shame, and fear, as the sixth component of this conceptualization of stigma. Andersen and colleagues (2022), in their analysis of the work of Link and Phelan, offer a simpler, more streamlined definition of stigma that requires labeling; negative stereotyping; linguistic separation (giving a name to the labeled difference); and asymmetry of power. The conceptualizations emphasize that stigma is best understood as a community and social-level phenomenon.

Stigma based upon an individual's HIV status results in adverse health and psychosocial outcomes (Perger et al., 2025; Wendt et al., 2025; Yigit et al., 2025). Manifestations of stigma comprise *enacted* stigma, including overt acts of discrimination, prejudice, and/or violence; *felt* (or *anticipated*) stigma, an individual's expectation they will experience a negative encounter or rejection due to their HIV status; and *internalized* (or *self-*) stigma, an individual's acquiescence to their stigmatized status and incorporation into their inner life and value system (Bagchi et al., 2019; Peltzer & Pengpid, 2019; Turan et al., 2017). Detrimental HIV stigma outcomes include disengagement from care, decreased ART adherence, increased substance use and rates of depression and anxiety, and social isolation (Earnshaw et al., 2013; Kota et al., 2023; Meyers-Pantele et al., 2022; Relf et al., 2021; Stangl et al., 2019). Since many PLWHA possess multiple, intersecting forms of stigma based on race, class, sexual orientation, and gender identity (to name just a few), their outcomes may be exacerbated (Jones et al., 2025; Kerr et al., 2022; Lancaster et al., 2022; Norcini-Pala et al., 2025). Despite medical advancements, HIV remains highly stigmatized. In 2024, 43% of adults held at least one stigmatized belief about PLWHA; this prevalence of stigma has increased from 31% in 2021 (Grasso et al., 2026). Approximately one-third of adults report fear of close contact with PLWHA (Grasso et al., 2026).

Participants shared how stigma affects their work with clients. They considered how they defined stigma and provided examples of addressing it. Participants also discussed the role of intersectional stigma. Finally, they revealed what their family, friends, and other community members thought about their work with PLWHA.

Defining Stigma

Participants consistently emphasized that stigma is a negative influence in their clients' lives. PLWHA remain subject to scorn and prejudice because of their diagnosis despite years of biomedical progress. Derek noted that stigma was omnipresent.

> But I mean, the stigma around it [HIV], in many ways, in many corners, is wild. It's a wildly, wildly stigmatized disease, and there's a lot of initiatives and education around there to sort of challenge that or say otherwise, but it's out there. It's very real. (Derek)

Derek's observation that stigma remains "very real" serves as a pointed rejoinder to narratives that downplay the ongoing significance of the epidemic and underscores that social burdens persist, independent of treatment advancements. He also pointed to the enduring nature of HIV stigma, suggesting that it may resist initiatives and educational efforts intended to mitigate its impact. As a PLWHA, Derek may be especially attuned to the persistence of stigma given his own lived experiences.

Tony's definition of stigma encapsulated both individual-level processes and discrimination and differential treatment at the community level.

> Being treated and judged based on your status and being treated differently whether it's with dating or having family members blame you for your status or not want to have physical contact or exclude you, and then also just like the outright discrimination from housing and jobs and things as well. But then also like the internalized stigma of feeling a lot of shame and self-blame around being positive. (Tony)

Tony's account highlights the persistence of outdated beliefs that frame HIV as dangerous and readily transmissible, reflecting how entrenched misconceptions continue to affect attitudes of the virus. They also linked internalized stigma to diminished psychosocial wellbeing, which has been observed in PLWHA (Pryor & Reeder, 2011; Van Der Kooij et al., 2021).

Like Tony, Billy viewed stigma as a denial of PLWHA's essential humanity: "And stigma is people looking down at or putting people in a box and deciding that you're this thing, you're this person, you are less than, you are somehow to be othered". The idea of "othering", in which PLWHA are positioned as abnormal and outside of the bounds of society, remains a central feature of how stigma is experienced (Logie, 2022; Rohleder, 2016; Silva-Brandao & Ianni, 2022). Participants noted that stigma was a substantial obstacle in their work with clients, affecting not only how clients understood their diagnosis but also how they engaged with care, relationships, and systems of support. Stigma is not a peripheral concern, but a central presence in the lives of PLWHA that requires social workers to develop skills to appropriately respond to this phenomenon.

Addressing Stigma

Programs and policies designed to address stigma and its impact on PLWHA require interventions at both the individual level and within the broader socioecological factors and systems that sustain and reproduce stigma (Ferguson et al., 2023; Pantelic et al., 2019; Relf et al., 2021). Given the limitations of their settings, available resources, and job responsibilities, participants' efforts to address stigma occurred mostly at the individual level. Luca recalled their practicum with an organization that sponsored a syringe access program. They revealed that clients who were not living with HIV would make inappropriate use of humor when discussing the virus. Luca observed the social construction of stigma in real time and struggled to respond in a compassionate manner.

> And I know people often will make jokes or try to make light of something when they're feeling uncomfortable. And there's a lot of that around HIV, especially people who are in treatment centers. Again, not to throw cis men under the bus, but a lot of cis men would make jokes because they were embarrassed that they didn't know something or again the fear of being considered queer or being perceived as queer in some way. Figuring out how to interact with those folks in a way that was empathetic, but very firm and clear, too, that that kind of joking isn't okay, and just perpetuates the stigma that's based on a lot of falsehoods. Yeah, that was a challenge, too, because I would just get really annoyed. I'm like, just stop. Just stop. Just shut up. I mean, I could say that, but it's not helpful to say that. (Luca)

Luca noted that HIV stigma was associated with a fear that individuals seeking services with their organization might be perceived as queer. Given the close relationship between queerness and HIV status, interventions to combat HIV stigma must also address intersecting homophobic attitudes and beliefs (Frye et al., 2017; Garcia et al., 2016). Joking, even when ostensibly delivered with benign intent, may have harmful effects on those with stigmatized identities (Horisk, 2024). In the initial stages of their social work career, Luca was tasked to find a balance between stopping disparaging remarks while not alienating clients—a difficult proposition for even the most skilled social worker.

Derek remembered an experience from his first-year placement when he disclosed his HIV status to intervene with a client with internalized HIV stigma. Self-disclosure of a stigmatized identity can be effective at addressing stigma, benefitting those who make the disclosure and those who receive the information (Ballinger et al., 2023; Frese, 2015;

Gjesfjeld & Kahn, 2024). Like Luca, Derek was working with individuals with substance use challenges. A straight man living with HIV shared his anxiety that he might infect his child through casual contact. Recognizing the client's internalized stigma, Derek made the spontaneous choice to reveal his serostatus.

> He said things like, he was unhoused and living [on the streets], but he did have a young son back where he's from and he's like, oh, you know, I'm afraid if I play ball with my boy that I'm going to give him HIV. So just, you know, he internalized a lot of sort of stigma and negative attitudes. So just to be able to be there and support him as somebody living with the virus, it was a really meaningful experience. (Derek)

As Derek gained more social work experience, his views on self-disclosure became more measured, though he continued to believe it could offer comfort to clients experiencing stigma. At the same time, he acknowledged uncertainty about whether his disclosure achieved the intended effect, reflecting an ongoing process of critical reflection and professional discernment in his practice.

Stigma manifested in August's younger clients with their medications. PLWHA often worry family members and/or roommates could discover their HIV medications. This may result in poor medication adherence and greater incidence of internalized stigma (Dworkin et al., 2019; Fisk-Hoffman et al., 2024; Zhang et al., 2025). Interventions to manage medication visibility and support adherence are crucial for the health of PLWHA. August shared that he suggested clients transfer their pills into more innocuous-looking bottles that would not raise suspicion.

> How do I figure out a way…so that they feel comfortable enough to take their meds or keep their meds in a place where they will remember to take it? How do I

> reduce the experience of perceived stigma or that somebody's going to find out something? Even having patients have an old or dump out a vitamin bottle and put their antiretroviral meds into a vitamin bottle, and that became like their daily vitamin, it felt like we were finding ways to reduce perceived stigma, or to reduce that feeling of perceived stigma so that they can just take care of themselves rather than addressing the reasons that stigma is there in the first place. (August)

August recognized that, in addressing stigma, he needed to support his clients with practical interventions, rather than tackling larger systemic issues that perpetuated the stigma. This orientation demonstrates a pragmatic approach where early career social workers learn to concentrate their energy on immediate supports while remaining cognizant of the broader structural forces that impact clients' lives.

Simon wrestled with addressing stigma in older clients who were unhappy with their physical appearance. Interventions aimed at improving body and image satisfaction among PLWHA are varied, including cognitive-behavioral therapy (Blashill et al., 2017), nutrition counseling and support (Feldman et al., 2011), weekly semaglutide injections to stimulate weight loss (Eckard et al., 2024), and dermal filler for the face (Carey et al., 2007). Some of Simon's clients experience sunken cheeks or increased abdominal fat fairly typical for older PLWHA; these physical changes served as constant reminders of their HIV status and advancing age. Simon felt constrained with what else he could offer these clients.

> Honestly, it's very hard. A lot of validation happens. I don't have an intervention for it aside from holding space and kind of just validating how they're feeling. I can't say, well, don't look in the mirror ever again, cover up the mirror. It's a...

> yeah, it's acknowledging that, yes, it must be hard to have this frequent reminder of this, you know, traumatic thing that you experience. And again, the trauma of it goes beyond just the diagnosis. It's just what all you experience during that time. (Simon)

Older PLWHA, a rapidly growing population, are faced with greater health and psychosocial challenges throughout the aging process (Crawford et al., 2023; Guaraldi et al., 2024; Pollak et al., 2025). Interventions that address HIV stigma in older PLWHA must account for how ageism and other forms of oppression complicate these efforts, while underscoring the need for early career social workers to develop an intersectional approach as part of their professional growth.

Intersectional Stigma

Intersectional stigma refers to the synergistic aggregation and interactions of multiple forms of stigma that create a distinct form of oppression (Logie et al., 2011; Sievwright et al., 2022; Turan et al., 2025). Individuals at most risk of acquiring HIV are often marginalized due to race, gender identity, and gender expression; PLWHA encountering multiple forms of stigma receive worse care and experience more negative health outcomes compared to those not similarly situated (Jackson-Best & Edwards, 2018; Karver et al., 2022; Watkins-Hayes, 2014). Participants observed how intersectional stigma harms their clients. T noted that their queer PLWHA clients had less social supports and greater challenges than their non-queer PLWHA clients.

> I would say the main difference in terms of challenges would be in terms of their support system, because in REDACTED, the queer community is a lot more discriminated against compared to other states. For the queer clients versus the

> non-queer clients, the non-queer clients would, even though their support system wouldn't be aware of their status, they would still be supportive of the person, but for the queer clients, many of them didn't have a support system or their support system was incredibly small and unable to really assist them with any additional challenges they may be having. (T)

T observed how homophobia is a critical element of oppression that negatively impacts queer clients. The suppression of sexual orientation, coinciding with fears of potential disclosure, can result in worse health outcomes for PLWHA who experience homophobia (Arnold et al., 2014b; Ramos et al., 2021). Early career social workers like T come to recognize that no single aspect of a client's identity can be understood in isolation. Understanding how multiple identities and experience interact and compound one another is an important professional developmental task.

Dan believed that HIV stigma and homophobia were closely related. He saw how some clients felt they deserved their diagnosis as punishment for their sexual orientation.

> I feel for a lot of the folks I'm working with, they're having HIV, it feels like an extension of challenges they're already dealing with just being queer. I'm working with a lot of Black and Brown patients. And so, this isn't like a common thing, but for a lot of folks, they're getting HIV is a really, I mean, this is really kind of sickening, but it's, there have been times where that's been presented as, well, you got what we knew you were going to get. They've gotten feedback from family, sometimes from friends. But yeah, I would say HIV feels like an extension of stigma they were already experiencing just from being queer and being in spaces that weren't as accepting or conducive of that. (Dan)

Davoudpour and colleagues (2025) argue the persistent association between HIV and perceived immorality, including queer sex, helps explain the enduring impact of HIV stigma.

Several of Ashley's clients are stigmatized for their sexual orientation and their use of substances and engagement with sex work.

> Part of the stigma for HIV is the idea that it's sexually transmitted, so, and also through IV use, so there's a moral component to it. Like, you're bad because you had unprotected sex, or you're bad because you did sex work, or you're bad because you're gay, or you're bad because you inject drugs. So that's the social stigma of it, and then also a lot of misunderstanding about it. (Ashley)

PLWHA who use substances report complex and layered forms of stigma that shape decisions about disclosure of HIV status, engagement with medical care, and the continued use of substances as a coping strategy (Lancaster et al., 2022; Levi-Minzi & Surratt, 2014; Stutterheim et al., 2016). Injection drug use, one of the primary routes of HIV transmission, is especially stigmatized, complicating interventions designed to address HIV among IDUs (Endres-Dighe et al., 2025; Weger et al., 2025). Sex work is also highly stigmatized, resulting in increased risk of HIV and barriers to effective treatment (Fitzgerald-Husek et al., 2017; Lyons et al., 2020; Yang et al., 2025).

Billy thought that intersectional stigma discouraged harm reduction efforts, such as syringe access programs, known to decrease HIV incidence (Kronfli et al., 2025; Packham, 2022; van Santen et al., 2023).

> You know, there's still a stigma attached to HIV because of the way it is spread. I think there's still a stigma for LGBT folks. I think there's still a stigma for drug

users. You know, our governments are not on our side anymore. And that's the federal government, but also our local government has done away, is doing away, trying to do away with needle exchange. Needle exchange saves lives. Needle exchange stops the spread of HIV. You're just going to have more HIV positive people. That's just messed up. (Billy)

Cities overwhelmed by substance use are rescinding their support of harm reduction efforts, arguing these programs enable addiction, promote hazardous behaviors, and place residents and neighborhoods at risk of crime and unsanitary streets (Whelan, 2024). Such responses may be understood as a displacement of stigma from individuals onto the services intended to support them, as well as the spaces where they gather (Tempalski et al., 2007). Interventions designed to address intersectional stigma can play a significant role in efforts to end the HIV epidemic and social workers must closely monitor and address the impact of intersectional stigma experienced by PLWHA (Rodriguez-Hart et al., 2022; Smith et al., 2022). Early career social workers should be equipped with skills and awareness to recognize how overlapping stigmas affect client engagement, access to care, and long-term health.

Community Responses

Participants were asked how individuals within their social networks reacted when they shared that they were working with PLWHA. There is little research that explores the perspectives of social workers' family and friends[9]. Participants reported that most individuals were supportive of their work, although there was the occasional awkward or insensitive interaction which suggested the presence of stigma. Winnie's family was encouraged by their new role, although their grandmother raised a concern.

> They think it's very cool. I will say when I told my grandmother last year, she was very confused and she was like, don't get HIV. And I was like, Nana, I'm not gonna sleep with my patients. Don't worry. And she was like, oh, okay. She didn't really get what I was doing, I think, but my family thinks what I'm doing is really cool and important and super aligned with what I have been saying I've been wanting to do. (Winnie)

Fear of contagion and misconceptions about routes and likelihoods of transmission persist, facilitating HIV stigma (Hughes & Alford, 2017; Kim et al., 2025; Peifer et al., 2025). While Winnie was born around the time ART was introduced, their grandmother's understanding of the epidemic was most likely influenced by memories of the nadir of the epidemic, emphasizing a generational divide in attitudes and beliefs about HIV.

Ashley revealed how her neighbor reacted when learning that she works with PLWHA.

> I used to have a mechanic who lived behind me, his shop was behind my apartment. And at some point, I mentioned that I work in HIV care. And he was like, oh, I'm gonna stay away from you, as if I was gonna give it to him. And I was like, I don't, first of all, I'm not HIV positive. Second of all, I'm not planning on sharing blood or bodily fluids with any of my patients. Like, I don't intend on doing any of those things. So just the misunderstanding of it. (Ashley)

She specifically connected her neighbor's stigmatized attitudes about HIV with a lack of information about the virus, which has been demonstrated to contribute to stigma (Pitasi et al., 2018).

While Jenny's family had no concerns with her work with PLWHA, members of her community were more apprehensive. Jenny, who identifies as Hispanic, noted that HIV stigma is prevalent among certain segments of this population. Latin/Hispanic PLWHA are often marginalized within their cultural communities (Felipe da Cruz et al., 2023; García et al., 2022). Jenny educated individuals in her social networks about the realities of HIV.

> Within my immediate family, it was normal. I think once I tell other individuals, they're like, oh, really? They get that reaction, or I get that reaction from them. And I think it's because of the stigma that exists, especially when I tell people within my culture, people get scared when they hear HIV or AIDS. I mention it, I always inform them about it and inform them that it's not, you know, it's not what they think it is or what the stigma is around this disease. And anyone can have it and that doesn't mean that they're any less of a human being just because they have a certain disease. (Jenny)

Bryan recalled frustration when their sister's boyfriend asked whether they were scared to work with PLWHA: "It's really funny. I had my sister's boyfriend ask me something about that. And I remember being kind of offended. I was just like, that's such a regressive view to be scared. It sort of feels childish, to be honest". Given that this individual was mostly likely a generational peer to Bryan, their attitude cannot be explained as evidence of a generational gap. Retrograde ideas and fears about HIV have not disappeared with the decline in the epidemic's lethality. The reactions of family, friends, and other individuals to participants' involvement with PLWHA, ranging from strong support to awkward comments to suggestions of avoidance, indicate that social workers must not only be vigilant about the role stigma plays in the lives of their clients, but also how it may affect their connections within their personal networks.

Conclusion

Community-level factors exert a significant influence on the experiences of PLWHA and social workers. The challenges participants reported in collaboration with outside providers suggest a need for innovations in inter-organizational communication and partnerships. Stigma, especially intersectional forms of this phenomenon, remains a barrier for PLWHA that affects health outcomes and engagement with social workers. Understanding and addressing these community-level factors require social workers to empower clients through individual interventions while working toward broader systemic changes and acknowledging how community conditions and stigma influence clients' health and wellbeing trajectories over the life course.

Chapter 8
Policy-Level HIV Governance

Policy and societal factors within the socioecological model influence the broader conditions that structure how early career social workers engage with PLWHA. These macro-level factors include federal and state laws, funding structures, public health priorities, and prevailing social attitudes and beliefs about HIV. Early career social workers learn that client outcomes are closely connected to the functioning of systems that seem far removed from the individual. Learning how these systems work together and against each other and understanding the issues that impede or facilitate client care are important social work skills and knowledge crucial for professional development. In this chapter, seven themes were identified: client concerns about current events; social worker concerns about current events; HIV as a matter of social concern; need for HIV-specific services and programs; development of systems awareness; HIV exceptionalism; and future of social work with PLWHA.

Client Concerns about Current Events

Interviews for this project commenced in December 2024, shortly after Donald Trump was elected to a second term as President, and concluded in April 2025, approximately three months into his administration. Within this relatively short time span, there were great upheavals and uncertainty regarding HIV policy on the national and international levels. Soon after Trump took office, the U.S. instituted a freeze on all foreign aid, effectively halting the distribution of HIV medication purchased with U.S.

funds to foreign countries (Mandavilli, 2025a). The highly regarded PEPFAR (President's Emergency Plan for AIDS Relief) program, which disburses billions of dollars to fight the epidemic across the globe, appeared at risk of dismantling (Taylor et al., 2025). The new administration paused all federal grants and loans, then seemingly reversed course days later, sowing confusion among individuals and organizations (Stein et al., 2025). The chaotic vagueness was especially concerning to PLWHA worried they could lose housing and medical care funded through federal grants (Dawson, 2025). In March 2025, the administration considered draconian cuts to the CDC HIV prevention budget and elimination of funding for EHE initiatives. While not constituting a formal budget request, these discussions demonstrated the administration's indifference to the needs of PLWHA and those at risk of infection (Dawson, 2025). Fear and uncertainty were not just the byproducts of these proposed changes and revisions; they were significant administrative tools designed to intimidate individuals and communities and enforce the agenda of the new President (Conyers, 2025; Wies, 2025).

Participants shared that clients were frightened by the developments emanating from Washington, D.C. Tony remembered facilitating a support group for PLWHA when members raised concerns that their health care might be in jeopardy.

> Like the day of the federal freeze, when I was running a support group and we kind of we talked together about how it might affect funding pretty immediately and encouraging people to fill their meds that day. And we were going to request samples and figure out ways to create more resources within our community directly. And then people ask me all the time about like, how is Ryan White or Medicaid or Medicare gonna be affected? And, or some folks are worried about

> targeted discrimination against folks who are positive. And so I think it does come up and it is definitely a big concern. (Tony)

Tony witnessed the stress of their clients and worked with their colleagues to develop innovative ways to ensure their clients could still access their medications if funding evaporated. This response shows how social workers learn to adapt in real time to policy uncertainty while maintaining continuity of care.

Winnie observed similar reactions among their clients who received medical case management.

> People have definitely been really worried, which makes sense. I know in my supervisions with my case managers every week, you know, case managers have been kind of talking about this, these same clients who have expressed continued fears over, just Trump in general or the agency losing funding or closing and there you know was like a hot second with the executive orders where we thought like oh, are we losing funding, are we all out of a job now? Do we have to stop case management? (Winnie)

Attending to these tensions would be challenging even for seasoned practitioners; for Winnie, they occur at the beginning of their career when clinical instincts are still forming. Navigating competing demands from clients, organizations, and changing policy landscapes requires early career social workers to tolerate ambiguity and act under conditions of uncertainty. Additionally, Winnie may need to address their own feelings about the broader political climate. Supporting clients while processing their own reactions highlights the complex affective labor often required of social workers.

Jenny shared her clients' fears that proposed changes would negatively impact their wellbeing. The political turmoil was viewed as an existential threat for who depend on federal assistance.

> Well, like I said before, a lot of our patients that are low income get medical insurance through Medicaid. And I know that that has been in discussions within topics of cutting funding for Medicaid, Medicare. And so we have gotten concerns from our clients of, what are we going to do if my Medicare gets cut off? Or what am I going to do if my Medicaid gets cut off? Like where am I going to get my medical care? How am I going to afford my medical care? How am I going to afford to eat or find or bring food to my house when my SNAP benefits may be cut off? (Jenny)

PLWHA experiencing scarcity and insufficiency of material resources, in conjunction with social instability, are known to have poorer health outcomes and chronic inequalities (Szychowiak et al., 2025; Whittle et al., 2020). Clients turned to their social workers for reassurance, but participants found themselves just as confused and uncertain.

Other participants stated their clients had a more sanguine perspective of current events. Paige believed her clients were indifferent to recent developments. She contextualized this lack of interest to her clients' histories of challenges: "a lot of my clients were just like, you know, same shit, different day. You know, they have been marginalized and oppressed for decades. So they're like, whatever". Paige understood that her clients' attitudes were based on a foundation of accumulated experiences with systems of care, and she used this insight to inform her social work practice. Similarly, Simon noted his clients are often more focused on matters of more immediate concern due to their precarious living situations.

> I think the folks that I'm working with currently, I think if they operate of like, you know, I'm aware of all this up here, but right now, you know, I'm here. I'm focusing on, you know, right now. I'm doing this and when it becomes a real issue per se, then I can address it. I think my folks right now, that's kind of how they operate. (Simon)

This orientation toward immediacy reflects how instability can narrow clients' focus, prioritizing day-to-day survival over abstract future-oriented concerns. Early career social workers come to recognize that the goals that they may initially identify may not agree with their clients' priorities.

Josh noted that one of his gay PLWHA clients voted for President Trump in 2024. While Trump improved his standing among several demographics, LGBT voters shifted away from the President (12%) in favor of his opponent, then Vice-President Kamala Harris (86%) (Egan, 2024). Josh believed that his client was in denial that he could lose his health care because of recent policy shifts.

> My older client is actually a Trump supporter. I think, you know, he's like, oh, I won't get affected by this. Like, you know, I don't want to say the cult, but he is one of those people that, you know, he doesn't think the leopard's gonna eat his face. He's like, oh, I voted for Trump. I'm a cis gay man. I'm upper middle class, like I won't have my medication taken away or it won't skyrocket to the roof in cost or, he does not talk about that at all. (Josh)

Josh's account demonstrates how clients' political beliefs may affect their perceptions of social vulnerability. For early career social workers, such moments require a careful and ethical balance of respect and critical awareness as they learn to support their clients without imposing their own beliefs.

Since the conclusion of data collection for this project, the HIV policy terrain has become more challenging. In July 2025, the One Big Beautiful Bill Act (OBBBA) mandated changes to Medicaid eligibility that may eliminate coverage for many PLWHA (International Association of Providers of AIDS Care, 2025). The Presidential Advisory Council on HIV and AIDS (PACHA) warned that proposals emanating from the U.S. House of Representatives could eliminate funding for domestic and global efforts to combat the epidemic, remove approximately $1 billion from the CDC's budget, and gut key parts of the Ryan White CARE Act (Peterson, 2025). States with significant budget deficits have restricted eligibility requirements for HIV drug assistance programs that serve as a last resort for low-income PLWHA; tens of thousands are at risk of losing access (Mandavilli, 2026). As the political wrangling continues, PLWHA and their social workers may find themselves working together to make sense of these developments.

Social Workers' Concerns about Current Events

Participants described an undercurrent of fear pervading their workplaces and interactions with clients. In the social and political environments in which social workers are expected to carry out their work, fear increasingly functions as a governing principle and a primary mechanism through which power is exercised (Remnick, 2025). Dan remarked how threats to funding produced a climate of anxiety for both clients and staff, as the possibility of losing resources unsettled the sense of stability on which care depends.

> I think there's talks around funding and fears around funding and concerns around what this could mean for patients. So…I do think there's been a fear that has kind of permeated that. Yeah, when you're in a space that is funded, it can feel really

scary of not knowing if that's going to be impacted or then it's connected that if your patients are going to be impacted or their capacity to get the medications they need are going to be impacted. (Dan)

Leo shared how their colleagues were coping with uncertainty. They relied upon their knowledge of systems, particularly funding sources, to assuage their anxiety.

> You know, right now in this current political climate and in this field of work that we do, everyone's terrified. So being someone who has an interest in understanding how funding works, not that I know a lot, you know what I mean? But I think that it has helped me keep like sort of a level head and not being just like totally panicked, you know, I don't know. But it's also scary, it's bad. (Leo)

Leo's assertion that "everyone's terrified" speaks to the emotional injuries that policy battles inflict upon PLWHA and their social workers. Already struggling with burnout and emotional exhaustion (Ratcliff, 2024), social workers engaged with PLWHA report heightened levels of stress. For early career social workers, who may be the least-tenured, lowest-salaried, and most burdened by debt in their organizations, the current atmosphere of fear may seem suffocating. Derek found it difficult to express his concerns for PLWHA and his own health. He drew on his knowledge of the epidemic's history to place the current moment in perspective.

> There's this wild sort of dissociative element to it because so much is happening and there's a lot of information around it, but I'm not sure the actual impact. But one thing I'll say is, you know, AIDS activists and AIDS workers had to fight so hard for the government to pay attention to this disease, you know, and to get funding to support us. And we have been amazingly successful in that…But then

to see the federal government just erase all the sort of digital imprint like on the internet, all the websites and it's really scary. It's like, oh gosh, what does that mean and will folks without private insurance be able to access their medication or folks that need help with their copays through private insurance or whatever be able to access their medication? I mean, you know, I'm one of them frankly…I mean it's really scary. You know, I don't quite know how to wrap my mind around it and I don't want to catastrophize and panic, but it feels really scary, you know. (Derek)

Derek's reference to dissociation suggests an effort to distance himself from the surrounding political discourse. His understanding of the current moment is shaped by a distinctive combination of personal experience and historical awareness not available to other participants. Derek contends with recent developments as both a social worker and as a member of the PLWHA community.

Paige also sought to shield herself from the tumult of current events until it became impossible to ignore.

> I've been trying to keep my blinders on, I don't want to engage in the discourse, like, ask me…about things that I can see in front of me every single day. But I, you know, we've gotten to a point where I can no longer ignore that blissfully, because our REDACTED funding was just cut. So we were a place where people could come just get a full bag of nutritious meals, nutritious microwaved meals made by chefs across the city. And we can't do that anymore. We were a place where homeless people could come get a hot meal, as long as we were open and that we're not allowed to do that. And we also had plans to hire a resource

> navigator, which is someone that works with REDACTED, or they did before that shut down. And they do all of our data collection for us to receive funding. And so now we're down one, things like that. But my bigger concerns are around cuts to Medicaid and Medicare. I don't think that my agency is going to close its doors. But I've worked for agencies that I thought that about that did close their doors.
> So who knows? I think that no matter what happens in the future, my clients are going to be fine. They'll find a way. (Paige)

Paige minimized any concerns for her own job security even as she acknowledged that her organization was losing staff and resources. Her optimism rested largely on her faith in the resilience of her clients, a quality she had observed repeatedly. It remains an open question whether individual-level resilience can adequately compensate for the potential loss of services and supports.

HIV as Social Concern

In 2025, the United States declined to commemorate World AIDS Day, which has occurred every December 1st since 1988 (Mandavilli, 2025b). Given the Trump Administration's apparent antipathy toward the epidemic, this snub was disappointing but not surprising (Blumenfeld, 2025). It sent an unmistakable message that, at least for those ensconced in the highest echelons of government, HIV is not worthy of recognition. However, this decision may also reflect a broader public consensus that regards the epidemic as history rather than a social and political present-day reality (GLAAD, 2024). Participants reflected on whether HIV is still regarded a matter of social concern and shared their observations about public attitudes and beliefs about the virus. Most participants felt the epidemic did not receive adequate public attention.

> It seems like it kind of waxes and wanes in social importance. I would say overall it's like not considered as important or not given the same kind of because it isn't currently like an epidemic or pandemic in the way that it was. But just because it is better doesn't mean that it is like good or that like we should stop paying attention to it. Yeah, I think it's not getting the attention that it needs. (Luca)

The transformation of HIV as "death sentence" to "chronic condition" was considered a critical factor in the decline in public interest in the epidemic. As the crisis abated and mass deaths receded from public view, so too did the sense of urgency that once made HIV a more visible social and political issue.

Emma recognized the epidemic is not finished, even if it does not command the same level of attention that it did during its most devastating years.

> People don't see it as like a death sentence anymore which is great. But yeah I think…more attention that is needed as far as like it being a social issue. I don't think it's talked about enough anymore. I think that there could be more attention around it for sure. Because…there's just like still so much work to be done. And especially with this like new administration, like it's just really scary what might happen. So I definitely think there's like a need for more, like a push for more. (Emma)

Emma welcomed that HIV is no longer perceived as a death sentence, yet she also worried that this shift has contributed to a diminished sense of urgency. Her comments suggest that reduced visibility should not be mistaken for resolution.

Tony stated that queer communities "have a lot more attention and appreciation for how HIV impacts people…but I think outside of the queer and trans community, no".

Similarly, Simon believed there is a divide between queer and non-queer communities concerning attitudes about the virus.

> I think certain communities care more than others. It may be more have some sense of it because, you know, the community may be, like the gay community, I imagine it may be more because it tends, you know, numbers are higher there. I don't think it's a social issue as it was during the epidemic, only because we aren't seeing these mass deaths from it or the impact of it. So in that sense, I guess I would say it's a social issue in the sense that…there's still stigma to it, all those things, but it's not a social issue in a sense where it's affecting the masses. (Simon)

However, even within queer communities, participants felt that generational location informs differing views of the scope and contemporary significance of the epidemic. Josh claimed there is a lack of awareness of HIV among younger people, unless they have been directly impacted by the epidemic.

> So many younger people are like forgetting almost that HIV exists or forgetting that these experiences happened, you know? These this epidemic happened, and this huge thing, and they're like, oh, it's all fine, it's all fine, like, HIV's not a big deal anymore, until someone gets it, and which people are still contracting…And so I think there's just this like, it's a big deal, but it's not a big deal. It's a big deal, but it's not a big deal. It's a big deal. And so I think that's what I see a lot with this younger client, is kind of like, I don't want to think about it, unless I really need to think about it. (Josh)

Most of the participants are members of generational cohorts that Josh asserted have forgotten HIV. These early career social workers came of age in a social and cultural environment in which HIV no longer occupied a prominent place in public life. When Josh stated, “it’s a big deal, but it’s not a big deal”, he expressed ambivalence, acknowledging that younger individuals are less educated about the virus and less familiar with PLWHA, compared to their older counterparts (Kaiser Family Foundation, 2017). Emerging social workers interested in working with this population must be prepared to counter forgetting, resist complacency, and introduce the realities of the epidemic to successive generations.

Billy, a long-time advocate for PLWHA, wondered who would carry HIV activism forward, given the relative indifference to HIV he observes among younger generations.

> I've had young LGBT folks say to me, they understand. No. You don't, you know, you don't, you don't know what it's like to have your best friend dying in front of you, wasting away into nothing, you know, cleaning the shit off of their legs. You don't, and I don't want them to experience that, right? I don't want them to go through that, but that, they have no idea, you know? And I, you know, “Tales of the City” did a recent, relatively recent incarnation. And there was a dinner party with a bunch of older guys and a young gay guy who said, well, I understand. And they shut him down. You know, like, you don't have any idea. And I felt for the boy, the young guy, but I also completely got it. Like, I agree, and I'm pissed about it too. And I really want young people to step up right now. Because you know, I could protest all day and then dance all night. I can't do that. I'm tired. I'm tired...I can't do it. I just can't, you know, and we need the young folks to step up and I don't know how to engage them, you know. I'm not on, you know, we've got to do some TikToks, you know, because they ain't on Facebook, I'll tell you that

much. (Billy)

Billy's account demonstrates that HIV has not necessarily lost its relevance, but that the epidemic is increasingly obscured by the passage of time and re-directed energies. For early career social workers looking to enter this field, the work demands they keep the needs of PLWHA in the public consciousness.

Need for HIV-Specific Services

Most participants worked in organizations or programs originally designed to address the specific needs of PLWHA. In the early years of the epidemic, HIV care was housed within specialized clinics and organizations due to the complex and rapidly changing understanding of the virus, the overwhelming need for psychosocial services and supports, and stigma and discrimination experienced by PLWHA in traditional medical and social service milieus (Cahill et al., 2015; Kimmel et al., 2016). PLWHA express a preference for specialized settings because of the relationships they developed with providers, cultural sensitivity demonstrated by providers, and competence and knowledge of providers (Granich et al., 2025; Lakshmi et al., 2018). However, there are compelling argument for mainstreaming HIV care into primary settings and organizations that are not HIV-exclusive. PLWHA often live with chronic conditions, such as diabetes and hypertension, that are more appropriately addressed within primary care settings (Bulstra et al., 2021; Goldstein et al., 2023). Integrated models of HIV and primary care have been demonstrated to have positive health benefits for PLWHA (Appenheimer et al., 2017; Edmonds et al., 2015; Pinto et al., 2024). Mainstream settings can make care feel less stigmatized when it is not explicitly connected to HIV (Steward et al., 2018). Furthermore, as the HIV care workforce decreases, specialized services will become overburdened as PLWHA live longer and become more engaged in care (Steward et al., 2020). Participants were asked whether there was still a place for specialized clinics and programs for PLWHA given the shifting landscape of HIV care. Participants acknowledged the medical and psychosocial needs of their clients could be met in different settings but worried this care would not be delivered in the same compassionate manner. Ashley noted that social workers who practice in specialty areas like HIV require familiarity with medical terminology and treatment options and cultural responsiveness to the needs of marginalized populations.

> There has to be a level of trans competence and like not being a homophobe. I mean, nobody working in healthcare should be anything phobic, but let's be real. I mean, so there's an additional layer of that, like we have to be extra socially conscious…But it's like, as a regular social worker, you can help people with HIV, but you have to also understand the language, the viral load and CD4 and, you know, the opportunistic infections, the Kaposi's sarcoma, that kind of stuff, like knowing the lingo, but that's also the case for any other specialty of social work…So there's the lingo, but I think not even just that. It's a specialty, but that there's like extra stuff. You need to be a certain kind of person to work in this population. (Ashley)

When Ashley referred to "extra stuff", she was pointing to the multiple identities, life circumstances, and stigmatized experiences PLWHA brings with them to the helping relationship. Social workers and other providers of care must possess the capacity to treat PLWHA with basic kindness and respect and strive to be, in Ashley's words, "extra socially conscious".

Billy believed that traditional social services organizations without a background in working with PLWHA would not be as responsive and affirming.

> I'm also grateful that those [HIV specialized] programs do still exist, and I will fight for them to continue to exist, because the populations that are being helped are populations that would really suffer to be seen and get served if they went completely away. Because the, you know, the straight housing services out there are going to look at a trans sex worker. Are they really going to go out of their way to help this person? You know, I mean, they might have to go by the numbers, but we know. Oh, I'm sorry, I lost your paperwork. Let's do it again. (Billy)

For Billy, ASOs and other organizations that serve PLWHA are irreplaceable and remain important sources of care, advocacy, and community.

Simon felt HIV care should be integrated into primary care settings. His observation illustrates how changes in the epidemic are closely implicated to questions of organizational viability and the future of HIV services.

> I think, you know, medically, scientifically, we know a lot more about HIV than we knew back in the 90s. We know how to manage it better. There are more options for medications around it. And I feel as though as numbers, I don't know what the current rates in terms of infections are every year, but I'm sure they have decreased than what they were way back when. So just looking from a straight business sustainability model, I don't know if you can sustain yourself on doing just that. And also by integrating into regular care, I think that also decreases the stigma as well. And so, yeah, I think, you know, the HIV federal dollars are also decreasing as well. (Simon)

Other participants were conflicted regarding the current need for specialized programs and services. Derek conceded most medical care could occur outside of HIV clinics but felt PLWHA would find mainstream provider interactions less supportive and culturally informed.

> I don't know, maybe both and? You know, I'm not sure. I've never been to just a medical provider, it's always been in a specialized HIV clinic and I just like knowing that they have, you know, special information and expertise with that, it's meaningful to me. But I think if one has wants to have like a more integrated care experience, PCP [Primary Care Physician], that's fine too. But one does have to be very careful, not just like in terms of medical knowledge, but sensitivity and sort of like cultural awareness around this. We're not gentle flowers, but there's a lot of potential for harm…I don't know. I think if people are going to be working with a sizeable contingent of folks living with this disease that a certain amount of medical, or sorry, specialized training is important. (Derek)

Derek's vacillation reflections the central tensions that define the debate about HIV-specific services. Medical providers often hold stigmatized attitudes about PLWHA and lack the latest information about the epidemic (Geter et al., 2018; Henny et al., 2019). HIV training modules and focused curricula, especially those that address intersecting issues such as stigma and substance use, have the potential to enhance care provision (Claborn et al., 2022; Wagner et al., 2025). If the integration of primary and HIV care is a goal, social workers, especially those entering the profession at this moment in the epidemic, must offer leadership and promote culturally appropriate programming and education to give providers the tools necessary to work with PLWHA.

Development of Systems Awareness

The socioecological model emphasizes that individual-level outcomes are intimately connected with macro-level forces that may appear far removed from the client. Participants demonstrated a solid understanding of the issues and challenges PLWHA experience and the systems, including governmental institutions and medical/social service infrastructures, that impact the delivery and quality of care. Several participants remarked they pursued social work because of its embrace of socioecological theories

> I had a job working in a group home and I didn't have any social work background…And it really introduced me to trauma in a larger picture, in ways that I hadn't really understood. Working with a lot of kids who experienced complex trauma and a lot of Black and Brown kids, a lot of queer kids. And I feel like I was kind of exposed to this other world that, you know, I know a little but not fully. And I wanted to understand more. I wanted to understand the systems. You know, I was seeing things after the fact, and I wanted to understand how to help kids cope, how to help, you know, kids thrive, and also, like, the systems in place, because everything wasn't there to support them. And I wanted to understand why and how, and how we could get more supports to them…Yeah, the bigger picture, I knew things were missing out of the equation. So that led me to getting my master's and trying to figure out all the systems in place that kind of work against folks but can hopefully try to change that. (Lynn)

Lynn's account highlights how socioecological approaches can draw people to social work by offering a framework that connects individual problems to the social and structural conditions that influence personal problems.

August learned that HIV care involves more than managing a virus; it also requires understanding the patchwork of policies and organizations that govern the everyday lives of PLWHA.

> I think that social work, because we are trained, or hopefully we are trained in the systems approach to care for people, that is going to be something that we are always challenging our colleagues who are more from the biomedical fields who don't get training necessarily in the social or the structural factors that can negatively impact care. I will say that HIV providers are some of the best in that area, compared with others I've interacted with from other specialties. I think that they know that they have to be aware of these other issues at the same time. And it's not as simple as here's the condition, treat it with a medication, send a patient on their way, like you might with a heart medication or a high cholesterol medication. Yeah, I think that there's a lot more nuance and I keep going back to intentionality for some reason, in depth to the level of care. (August)

When August referred to nuance and intentionality, he recognized that social workers engaged with PLWHA must be especially attuned to the multiple and intersecting factors that influence clients' health and wellbeing.

Vanessa stated that social workers must also address mezzo-level systems, including families and personal relationships, when working with PLWHA.

> I would say learning how all forms of life ultimately affects the person, so like all systems, so like social systems, government systems, their personal relationships, their family, just how overall, all the systems, how they, because in social work practice, we're taught how to be able to distinguish a person…seeing the person,

> working for the person, and just seeing how all the systems in play could affect the person. So that way you can help them overall and not just one part of the area. (Vanessa)

Most participants explicitly connected their work with clients to the legal, political, and economic systems that sustain care and affect their continued employment in this field. In doing so, they demonstrated commitments consistent with the socioecological model and the core values and ethical principles of the social work profession.

HIV Exceptionalism

HIV exceptionalism refers to the idea that HIV is distinct from other health conditions and warrants a unique response because of its early scientific uncertainty, high rates of mortality, and the stigma and discrimination associated with it (Smith & Whiteside, 2010). Demands that HIV be considered a political, social, and scientific priority, often to the exclusion of comparable health issues, resulted in research innovations, policy interventions, and dedicated funding that represented significant turning points in the trajectory of the epidemic (Daskalakis, 2025). However, exceptionalism led to onerous written consent laws for testing, statutes that subject PLWHA to criminal liabilities for having sex with others even with no risk of transmission, and surveillance systems that undermined individual autonomy (Bayer et al., 2017; Benton & Sangaramoorthy, 2021; Hoppe & Hall, 2025). Continuing to treat HIV as unique may perpetuate the stigma and discrimination that exceptionalism was meant to combat (Blain et al., 2021). But the "normalization" of HIV, or treating the virus similar to other chronic and manageable conditions, may obscure the stigma and barriers to care that PLWHA continue to experience (Villalba et al., 2025). Even with the considerable progress in HIV treatment, specialized programs and policies offer a level of care not yet available in traditional medical and social service settings (Ginossar et al., 2019; Hatcher, 2020). The debate over HIV exceptionalism suggests a potential middle road approach where antiquated policies are dismantled while programs and organizations that focus specifically on the needs of PLWHA are preserved (Hindmarch & Orsini, 2022).

Participants were asked whether HIV should still be considered exceptional or addressed like other chronic medical conditions. Most participants believed the history of the virus, the marginalized identities and experiences of those who live with it, and the stigmatized methods of transmission combine to make a case in favor of exceptionalism. August felt HIV was exceptional and addressed conditions of oppression that harm PLWHA.

> Yeah. I think it is, because I think it's been politicized in a lot of ways. I think the communities who are most impacted by HIV, Black and Brown communities, the queer community, they experience, I think, a level of marginalization, I don't know why this word's coming to my mind, but like demonization from certain political ideologies or people that perpetuate this stigma associated with HIV. So I think in a lot of ways, yeah, I think HIV is exceptional, that there needs to be intentional care and concern for not just the biomedical component of HIV, but the social, the structural, and the systemic levels that are very much present when working from a biomedical space. (August)

In calling for HIV to continue to enjoy special status, August explicitly centers this belief not on the medical aspect of the virus but rather on the continued discrimination that PLWHA experience. His use of “demonization” is striking, suggesting an intense form of stigma unlike other forms of oppression. Social workers engaged with PLWHA may, for the first time, understand that while the epidemic has changed for the better in many ways, clients still endure life challenges associated with their diagnosis. This first-hand knowledge may persuade social workers that HIV still demands exceptional approaches.

Other participants believed any discussion of HIV exceptionalism required some acknowledgement of the considerable gains in treatment resulting in better health outcomes for PLWHA. In Scott’s work with homeless individuals, he understood that while the history of the virus may be distinctive, the contemporary disease profile was not so remarkable as to require exceptional approaches.

> I think if you were to consider the history of HIV/AIDS and the epidemic, you would say it's absolutely distinct, a category of its own. I think for someone who's strictly looking at the experience of living with it, without reference to the history, you would say it looks like a chronic health condition that can be managed fairly well for decades even, and that there's significant momentum to work towards very improved methods of preventing it, treating it, and potentially even curing it. So I think it's hard for me to say that it appears to be just another chronic condition now because of the history, but the reality of it seems to be that the experience of working with people living with HIV and AIDS was that to them it was a chronic condition that they were managing. When someone would disclose they have HIV we would not experience a sense of alarm. We would just make a note, okay they have HIV. Are you seeing a doctor? Yes. Great…So it really just seemed like

another chronic condition, all things considered. (Scott)

Scott's reflection encapsulates the tension between HIV's historical exceptional status and its present-day clinical reality. For early career social workers, making sense of this challenging issue is a part of their professional development, particularly as they learn to position HIV within broader health and social service systems without losing sight of its significance.

Josh also recognized a disconnect between virus' history and its present day meaning. Josh's answer to the question of whether HIV should still be considered exceptional offers a fascinating summary of the larger debates surrounding this issue.

> I don't know. Some part of me wants to say yes, it's just another chronic medical condition at this point. But I am of a generation that's in the middle where, you know, I think millennials in general, PrEP didn't exist when I was coming into, I came out late, so I didn't come out until I was 26. PrEP still didn't exist, it started to exist in my, my early mid-30s…And so, I've lived with, had sex with, been in a community with a lot of people who survived the worst of that experience, you know, that epidemic. And it's hard for me to just think of HIV as another chronic health condition. And I also think…it's another chronic health condition as long as you have money and have health insurance…I think if I just sit still and look at it, if I just look at the elders in my life who've been through this terrible thing that happens, it doesn't feel like that, but when I, as I just say all this stuff out loud to you...So yeah, I guess I have a hard time reckoning with that, but yeah, it feels like in a lot of ways just another chronic health condition, at this juncture right now. I can say just right now in this time, that's what it maybe feels like. (Josh)

For Josh, the question of HIV exceptionalism is inseparable from his queer identity and experiences within queer communities during a pivotal time in the epidemic marked by the introduction of PrEP. His account demonstrates how generational positionality informs the ways early career social workers continue to make sense of the virus.

Derek understood that efforts toward normalization of the virus could substantially benefit PLWHA.

> Yeah, I've sort of thought about this question a lot, and in one way, in terms of messaging and challenging stigma, it's important to normalize it in that way or just lump it in with these other chronic medical conditions. That it’s manageable, no big deal. There’s a value in that. It's less complicated for me to say this as someone living with the virus, because there's a certain political utility to normalizing it. (Derek)

However, given his familiarity with the virus and history of activism, Derek asserted that HIV occupies a category of its own, a status that carries both benefits and drawbacks.

> But my emotional experience to that is of course it's not. Like, of course it’s not. There’s this insanely complicated cultural discursive history, it's meant so many things. And there's a negative component to it and there's a positive component to it. The negative is, you know, I don't know, it’s a really stigmatized condition, associated with irresponsibility, deviancy, all this sort of judgment, over-determined in that way, and to hold all those things is really impactful and painful. And just the fact that it's a disease that you could transmit, so that like makes it so much more different than say diabetes or whatever, because there's like, you know,

> when you get diabetes, the health department doesn't contact you and insist on, you know, heavily lean on you to disclose all your sexual partners or who you share drug paraphernalia with…You know, I belong to this collective called REDACTED and it's just like network of like artists and activists and AIDS workers, you know, positive and negative folks that do like art projects and have like, we had a meeting yesterday and just like, you know, for like support and chatting and it's like, amazing and beautiful, meaningful part of my life. You know, I've done, I made these films, I've done research, I built community, I've been able to teach. So because of this rich sort of cultural lineage that say like, diabetes doesn't necessarily have, there's a lot of ways to engage with it. So the stigma and the sort of negativity begets community and culture as a response. There's not many diagnoses that have it as such an identity that's burgeoned behind them. I would say, you know, substance use recovery is another one that has a rich history and I'm lucky to have both of them, right? So the stigma begets something in response, which is much more generative and positive. So by normalizing you're also sort of discounting that in a way, you know. (Derek)

According to Derek, if exceptionalism perpetuates stigma, normalization is not necessarily the panacea. Derek has thrived personally and professionally through his association with a community forged by HIV's unique historical, social, and medical status. Whether efforts to normalize the virus would be an existential threat to programming, services, and culture remains unknown. As treatments for the virus and demographics of the PLWHA community continue to evolve, social workers and other helping professionals will continue to debate HIV exceptionalism.

Future of Social Work with PLWHA

Participants were asked to predict the future of social work with PLWHA. Given the turbulent political environment when these interviews were conducted, it is not surprising that participants questioned the survival of programs and organizations dedicated to PLWHA. The uncertainty of the moment also made prognostication challenging for participants. Emma specifically cited the chaos emanating from Washington, D.C. when considering the future of social work with PLWHA.

> Right now, I really don't know. I think it's a scary time. I don't know what kind of funding cuts might like threaten this type of field. So that's concerning. I hope it continues to grow, but yeah, I definitely have concerns with the current political climate. (Emma)

For early career social workers like Emma who are trying to establish themselves professionally, the miasma of fear may lead them to reconsider whether social work with PLWHA is a sustainable career choice.

Josh agreed with Emma's assessment, adding that they were concerned that PLWHA could lose their access to life-preserving medications.

> I don't know…we're at just a weird moment in time with the political where it's like, we could go in any direction. I feel it could, the medication could disappear, become more difficult to get. Yeah, so I don't know. It's very confusing. (Josh)

Although the idea that medication access could simply vanish might seem fantastical or overblown, Josh gave voice to a very real anxiety affecting both clients and social workers.

Nora was also worried about the future of social work with PLWHA. She was aware that funding from the federal government did not just cover medical expenses but also supported essential psychosocial supports critical to the long-term health and wellbeing of PLWHA. Her answer reflected a pessimistic perspective.

> I mean, my hope is that the powers that be, I guess the federal government, still sees value in funding directed at this, at HIV programming, like Ryan White funding specifically. Yeah, my fear is that because, again, it's just a condition now, you know, that will go away, but that funding is being used for more than just the medical aspect...We have transportation through Ryan White funding. We have rental assistance through Ryan White funding. All that programming is really valuable. And so my hope is that it will continue. You know, we've lost, we used to have a housing program, at least in this county. Under Ryan White funding that is now gone. My hope is that those things will come back, but I'm not optimistic. And that's, again, that's a me thing. I don't operate from optimism. (Nora)

Simon stated that, given the trajectory of the epidemic, the social work field must adjust accordingly. While he was uncertain of what changes might be necessary, he surmised his role could become redundant.

> I do think that, and maybe this is on a larger scale, because HIV is not what it once was, at the height of the epidemic...I think we have to adapt and kind of recognize that, okay, while we see HIV is still present, it's not what it was, so how do we, you know, how do we deliver services? How do we survive as an agency? I mean, I'm not thinking more organizational, but I think it's, you know, our role, you know, our role is going to change. I may not be just an HIV social worker anymore because that population, you know, needs have shifted. People living with it, they aren't dying. They aren't dying from it any longer, per se. So, you

know, it's kind of, you know, while these values are important, how do I adapt to the current, you know, what's happening with it? (Simon)

Simon contemplated the potential end of his career as a social worker engaged with PLWHA. For early career social workers entering the field at this time of the epidemic, this uncertainty may be especially consequential, adding pressure to decisions about professional identity and specialization.

Ashley also acknowledged that advancements in HIV care could result in job loss. But while the treatment of HIV may change, underlying issues of oppression and marginalization still require enduring vigilance and support.

> I mean, it depends. It really depends because I was thinking about it and the EHE is Ending the HIV Epidemic. And it's like, if we end the epidemic, I don't have a job. But at the same time, that's what we want, to make people live longer and things like that. However, the funding is a huge thing right now. So I always keep in the back of my mind that federal funds are not the only funds. So REDACTED has money, the state has money, just because something's not federally subsidized doesn't mean that it won't be. I think that's just me being optimistic, like silly me and being positive. The future of HIV and social work, I think, I think as it becomes easier to medically manage it, we have Biktarvy and Cabenuva, I think the medical side will be easier. But I don't think that the poverty and the stigma, the transphobia, the homophobia, I don't think that's going away anytime soon. So I think there's going to be a need for us to be involved. (Ashley)

Ashley recognized that for PLWHA, their diagnosis is just one element, albeit an important one, in the constellation of challenges they encounter on a daily basis. While

PLWHA have better treatment options for HIV, they remain worse off physically, mentally, economically, and socially compared to their peers not living with the virus. If the epidemic were to end today, PLWHA would still need social workers.

Participants' projections of the future of social work with PLWHA were intertwined with their own professional identities. Early career social workers are caught in a bind, learning how to practice in this area while confronting the possibility that the work could change dramatically or even disappear. Although the future of social work with PLWHA is unknown, participants revealed that the structural forces and policy decisions that impact their clients' wellbeing also influence their professional trajectories.

Conclusion

This chapter demonstrates how policy and social contexts shape social workers' engagement with PLWHA and how they think about the virus itself. Medical advancements, dramatic shifts in the political climate, and threats to systems have raised concerns about the continued survival of services and organizations that have long supported PLWHA. Social workers are a mediating presence between individual clients and complex systems. Situating the findings of this chapter within the socioecological model demonstrates the necessity of interventions that extend beyond individual-level practice and for supports that sustain and uplift social workers navigating difficult and ever-changing terrain.

Chapter 9

Discussion, Implications, and Limitations and Strengths

Informed by the socioecological model and life course theory, this chapter answers the research question, "What are the experiences of early career social workers engaged with PLWHA?", through an analysis of the associations between and among individual meaning-making, interpersonal relationships, organizational and community contexts, and the broader structural and policy environments that frame social work practice. Across the narratives of participants, three interconnected themes emerge revealing how social work professional identity formation occurs through ongoing negotiation between rewarding and taxing work and institutional and societal supports and constraints. These themes include: making meaning of HIV; social work practice in the shadows of uncertainty; and HIV as a social work lens. The themes reveal social work practice as a dynamic interplay of self, systems, and society. This chapter reflects upon the study's implications for social work education, practice, research, and policy. Finally, limitations and strengths of the project are addressed.

Making Meaning of HIV

Throughout the study findings, HIV appears as a historically charged, emotionally complex, and socially mediated phenomenon that early career social workers continually interpret while taking into account the needs of clients, challenging organizational settings, shifts in public policy, and the historical legacy of the virus. Most participants

had only a rudimentary understanding of HIV prior to working with PLWHA. They conceded their knowledge was often based on outdated high school curricula or depictions of the virus filtered through the lens of popular culture. With a few exceptions, participants are members of generational cohorts that only know HIV as a chronic and manageable condition. Their understandings of HIV stand in contrast to the experiences of clients, especially those who lived through the worst years of the epidemic. Learning how HIV functions and appears in the body and the importance of markers such as viral loads and CD4 counts revealed to be an important social work task, but this education was not restricted to the virus' biomedical presentation. Participants discovered that HIV has a range of social, cultural, and political meanings that are highly context-specific.
They described how they were introduced to the persistence of stigma, the crushing weight of structural inequalities, and the resource-dependent, labor-intensive nature of the social work that helps keep PLWHA alive. Participants often suggested that HIV is no longer considered a significant social concern, a perception partly informed by their generational perspectives. Yet through their social work practice with PLWHA, they recognized that HIV and the meanings attached to it are deeply consequential for clients' health and wellbeing.

While participants understood that HIV is now considered a chronic condition, the findings suggest something more complicated. The virus may be manageable, but it remains *unresolved*. In other words, the incredible medical developments that have altered the trajectory of the epidemic have not eliminated the systems of oppression and conditions of deprivation that allow the virus to persist. New infections continue to occur, complicating narratives that the epidemic has been successfully settled. Most clients were described as engaged in care and generally adherent to medication regimens. However, participants shared how clients' experiences with mental illness, substance use, and complications related to aging confounded vigilance of their HIV health. Clients facing inadequate housing, limited transportation, food insecurity, and social isolation often struggled to maintain care. Participants, especially those engaged in medical case management, conceptualized their work as having two distinct but intersecting aims—addressing the medical aspects of HIV and attending to the social determinants of health impeding successful management of the virus. Social workers engaged with PLWHA learned that society has not kept pace with advances in HIV treatment, and this gap becomes the central reality affecting how they interpret and respond to clients' challenges. For participants, making meaning of HIV required a reconciliation of biomedical optimism, social and political disengagement, and the enduring structural inequalities that leave the epidemic fundamentally unresolved.

Discourses concerning the chronicity of HIV obscure the continuing impact of the virus and affect how social workers come to understand HIV. Several participants downplayed the significance of HIV and suggested it was not a salient issue in their clients' lives. In a list of client concerns, participants often ranked HIV near the bottom. They shared how their work primarily focused on clients' other health and/or material conditions, not on HIV care. However, when asked whether HIV should be considered exceptional or just another chronic condition, most participants asserted the virus is profoundly different from other health concerns because of its complex social history, persistent stigma, and the marginalized identities possessed by many PLWHA. Furthermore, participants were mostly in agreement that PLWHA still benefit from specialized services and programs. The findings demonstrate that early career social workers, in making meaning of the virus, wrestle with difficult contradictions about the past, present, and future of the epidemic. Participants confront these issues at a formative stage of their career development when their knowledge base and theories of practice are not fully formed. Unsettled disagreements about the continued relevance of HIV exceptionalism and movements toward normalization within policy and social service circles offer credence that HIV, for all the advancements in treatment, remains an unresolved condition.

Social workers must resist compartmentalizing HIV as a concern separate from the other challenges impacting clients' lives. The mental, physical, and social conditions of inequality harming their clients are the same conditions facilitating HIV transmission throughout the course of the epidemic (Watkins-Hayes, 2019). The virus' status as chronic and manageable requires a range of supporting conditions, including access to medications, the ability to store and consume pills safely, the mental and physical wellbeing required to make appointments and complete paperwork, and sufficient personal stability and security (King, 2021; McGrath et al., 2014). The book review and findings suggest the sustainability of these essentials is precarious. Once dependable streams of government funding are drying up. Participants shared that their organizations discontinued services and rescinded offers of employment. Social workers strained to find adequate resources for their clients. HIV is only chronic under carefully coordinated conditions of uninterrupted care, strong administrative capacity, stabile resources, and political will. If the safety net continues to weaken, the progress in the fight against HIV is at risk. Any regression in the course of the epidemic would likely come as a shock to participants whose only frame of reference has been one of uninterrupted progress. Chronicity is not a stable state that should be taken for granted, but a hard-fought achievement that remains conditional.

The unresolved nature of HIV means that social workers must gain the skills and knowledge needed to serve clients who continue to be viewed as morally suspect and dangerous, even when their viral loads remains undetectable. Participants stated how clients fear disclosure, even decades after their diagnosis, worried they would be rejected by family, ostracized by friends and neighbors, and denied employment and housing. Stigma remained a powerful presence in the lives of clients, even if their health was under control. The findings demonstrate that PLWHA are subjected to heightened monitoring and documentation that belies the belief that the virus is normalized. The crisis era of the epidemic ended years ago, but the afterlife persists. Early career social workers engaged with PLWHA must address the legacy of HIV and all its contradictions and complications to best serve clients while developing their professional knowledge, skills, and identities.

Because HIV is unresolved, any meaning-making of the virus must be tentative and open to reinterpretation. Participants observed very different attitudes and beliefs about HIV depending on their clients' generational positioning. Older clients, especially those who experienced the worst of the epidemic, survived years of death and despair and live with physical reminders of their diagnosis. Older PLWHA face questions about long-term care, financial insecurity, and an accumulation of health challenges. Younger clients with more recent diagnoses worried about dating and sex, and were connected to care more quickly than people from earlier generations. Participants noted that encounters with younger PLWHA were more transactional, while older PLWHA desired close helping relationships. Stigma was less of an issue for younger PLWHA compared to long- term survivors. Participants' accounts throughout the findings at all levels of the socioecological model demonstrate a wide variation of meanings of HIV often contingent on the identities and experiences of their clients. The unresolved nature of HIV forces social workers to explore their own beliefs and biases to ask: What does HIV mean to me? What does HIV mean for this client? What does HIV mean for my organization, community, and society? These questions, ideally discussed in supervision, can offer a helpful framework for early career social workers who are learning to locate their practice at the intersection of personal values, client experiences, and structural conditions.

The above questions are designed to prompt discussion of issues that are often minimized or discounted. Silence keeps HIV unresolved. Participants believed younger generations to be less knowledgeable and perceived little concern about the virus from the public. "Silence=Death" was a rallying cry for ACT UP. As HIV is less prominent in public discourse, meanings of HIV from previous generations are left undisturbed, casting a long shadow that threatens to eclipse present-day concerns of PLWHA. Social workers must contest antiquated ideas about HIV and resist the temptation to equate chronicity with resolution.

As social workers make meaning of HIV, they come to understand that the virus exists in multiple temporal dimensions simultaneously. Participants lauded biomedical innovations such U=U and the uptake of injectable ART that augur an end of the epidemic, but grappled with the possibility that this bright potential future may fail to materialize because of the vagaries of recent policy decisions. Funding instability portends a present where participants are confronted by structural and organizational stagnation that threaten their work environments and the wellbeing of clients. Several participants shared how clients' previous experiences with stigma and loss resonate today, emphasizing that the past is still very much alive. Social workers practice amidst a series of tensions where hope, uncertainty, and history coexist, shaping how they understand HIV, the needs of PLWHA, and social work's continued role in responding to the virus.

The findings of this study suggest that making meaning of HIV is not a one-time task, but an ongoing professional process through which early career social workers construe HIV's significance for clients, organizations, and society, while holding both biomedical optimism and persistent social inequities without fully resolving the tensions between them. Early career social workers must also account for the legacies of loss and stigma that have defined the past, present, and future of the epidemic. Meaning making is an act of interpretation that establishes the boundaries and expectations of social work practice.

Practice in the Shadows of Uncertainty

Early career social workers engaged with PLWHA practice within persistent conditions of uncertainty that span unpredictable shifts in policy, threats to organizational stability, and vicissitudes of client wellbeing, affecting their work and place within the social work profession. Uncertainty is properly understood not as an aberrant "bug" in the system, but rather a feature of social work practice impacting client experiences and encounters. Brashers (2001) defines uncertainty as "situations [that] are ambiguous, complex, unpredictable, or probabilistic; when information is unavailable or inconsistent; and when people feel insecure in their own state of knowledge or the state of knowledge in general" (p. 478). Todd and colleagues (2021) organize uncertainty into four broad categories: uncertainty as to the nature of the presenting problem; uncertainty as to the ethical course of action; social worker-based uncertainty, including self-doubt and disorientation; and relational uncertainty, related to perceived deficiencies in communication and intercultural understanding. While these conceptualizations may provide useful to social workers dealing with uncertain clinical encounters, they fail to adequately address the circumstances experienced by participants.

The findings of this study show that early career social workers engaged with PLWHA experience uncertainty at every domain of the socioecological model. At the individual level, participants shared how their social work education failed to prepare them for practice, while supervision in practicums could be inconsistent and inadequate. Participants felt powerless to address clients' health, material, and social challenges, exacerbated by a lack of organizational support during a critical time in their professional development. Experiences of uncertainty during this early stage of practice may carry greater weight for early career social workers still arriving at an understanding of the profession.

Policy disruptions left both clients and participants fearful about the continued availability of life-sustaining resources and the long-term viability of services. Insufficient organizational responses, coupled with uneven supervisory experiences and gaps in inter-organizational collaboration, failed to reassure participants during challenging moments. Early career social workers struggle to help their clients when armed with incomplete information and imprecise direction. Uncertainty generated by political actors trickles down to social workers, leaving them the burden of providing help when larger systems are actively discouraging, discounting, and demeaning care. The findings across chapters emphasize that uncertainty is a systematically generated practice context that shifts social work from responsive assessment and intervention to continuous exigency management, prioritizing risk mitigation and containment over planned, stable, and forward-looking forms of care.

Participants could not eliminate uncertainty but developed a range of strategies to mitigate its effects. These interventions demonstrated that the onus of systemic uncertainty often falls squarely upon the shoulders of early career social workers doing their best on behalf of clients. Participants addressed uncertainty through the use of cognitive reframing, remembering that service instability and resource insufficiency were systemic matters not indicative of personal inadequacy. Rather than worry about outcomes outside of their control, participants acknowledged their limitations and focused on their relationships with clients. Several participants explicitly drew upon their social work education and understanding of the socioecological model as guidance. For early career social workers, learning how to situate their work in broader contexts as a coping mechanism represented an important task of their professional development. Cognitive reframing was closely connected to other strategies for addressing uncertainty, such as limiting exposure to policy discourse, news reports, and speculative conversations with colleagues until the impact of changes was more comprehensible. This narrowing of attention demonstrated adaptive avoidance, allowing participants to continue functioning in difficult practice environments (Hofmann & Hay, 2018).

Other participants explained that the sharing of information and collegial relationships helped manage uncertainty. Participants in organizations that emphasized open and honest communication were grateful for this outreach, even when employers did not possess all relevant facts. Other participants noted that an understanding of funding systems provided them confidence that programs would not suddenly vanish and that multiple mechanisms could potentially sustain services for clients and their employment. Knowledge, even if imperfect and tentative, reduced emotional turmoil and restored a sense of agency for participants.

Another strategy to address uncertainty was reliance on relationships with clients and colleagues. When policies shifted, funding came under attack, or systems failed to respond to the needs of clients, participants leaned into relationship as a force for stabilization. Participants emphasized their personal presence and availability to clients when specific outcomes were beyond their control. They listened and validating concerns when clients expressed fears about the fate of the programs that were literally keeping them alive. For participants fortunate enough to experience strong supervision and organizational leadership, friendly relationships offered empathetic grounding and encouragement. During trying times, relationship was a protective factor for both participants and clients.

The reliance on relationship was critical to participants' development as social workers. Participants described how showing up for their clients, remaining engaged despite outside noise, and cultivating trust comprised effective and ethical practice despite disappointing or inchoate outcomes. However, some participants noted that relational work can take a heavy toll, leading to fears about incompetence, burnout, and disengagement. Relational engagement shifts responsibility from organizations and policymakers onto individual workers and raises concerns about the continued sustainability of this strategy. The findings of this study suggest uncertainty is not incidental to social work practice but fundamental to how early career social workers come to understand who they are and what the work demands of them and formative of the professional identities they carry throughout their careers.

HIV as a Social Work Lens

HIV appears as a lens through which early career social workers begin to make sense of the profession and their place within it. Participants entered practice with limited understandings of HIV, its complex history, contemporary biomedical advancements, and present social realities. Through their work with PLHWA, they recognized how individual health outcomes are affected by the interaction of structural inequality, social neglect, organizational capacity, and policy decisions, and how social work practice operates at the intersection of these socioecological factors. HIV facilitated professional socialization, where early career social workers learned not only what HIV is, but what social work demands: sustained socioecological approaches, relational labor, ethical decision-making under conditions of uncertainty, and engagement with systems that routinely fall short of clients' needs. This work took place at an important developmental stage of participants' careers, suggesting that early experiences with PLWHA may have lasting implications for their future social work practice. As the findings indicate, HIV served as a site where structural forces shifted from theoretical constructs to visible and real conditions, professional values were forged within the crucible of practice, and the work of becoming a social worker began in earnest.

Participants frequently described their journey to the social work profession as motivated by their desire to help others and address social injustice. In choosing social work, participants were motivated by the values and history of the profession, its socioecological orientation, and previous positive encounters with social workers. Most participants did not enter social work looking to engage with PLWHA specifically, but they found the work highly rewarding even in the most challenging situations. Through sustained involvement with clients and the systems designed to support them, they understood that conditions which make social work with PLWHA difficult were also those that emphasized the demands of practice.

Participants' engagement with PLWHA illustrates how core social work values and ethical principles are learned through enactment rather than formal instruction. Commitments to social justice and service were demonstrated as participants confronted the structural impediments that threatened to undermine their clients' care. Through sustained efforts within confounding policy and organizational environments, participants upheld the dignity and worth of their clients and embraced the importance of human relationships. Entering their roles with limited knowledge of HIV, participants learned the significance of competence, not just an ethical principle, but as a critical response to client needs. Together, the findings show how social work practice with PLWHA provided foundational early career experiences where values and principles were developed, tested, and performed within the socioecological framework.

Several participants acquired a strong comprehension of the socioecological model through their work with PLWHA, appreciating how individual health and wellbeing is embedded within larger systemic interactions. While some participants arrived at their practicum placement or job site with a general understanding of social determinants of health, their engagement with PLWHA compelled them to translate conceptual awareness into practical applications. Participants shared how they learned the importance of biomedical markers of the virus in tandem with the health, material, and social challenges that threatened to derail clients' progress. They learned that individual behavior could not account for client outcomes in isolation, thus reinforcing the theoretical underpinnings of the socioecological model.

At the levels of the individual and interpersonal, participants learned how to support and advocate for clients who were motivated and knowledgeable about their care yet negatively impacted by precarious living conditions and histories of stigma, discrimination, and maltreatment. The formation of relationship, as both ethical imperative and essential intervention, served as one of the most important tools participants relied upon to mediate clients' access to care and resources. At the organizational level, participants gained critical experience navigating fragmented systems and agency dysfunction on behalf of PLWHA. Participants were further exposed to community and policy contexts and described how instability from the federal government threatened to disrupt services and restrict access to medications and medical care. By incorporating socioecological perspectives into their efforts on behalf of clients, participants developed theories of practice that inform their professional development.

While early career social workers are socialized into the profession in a variety of settings and areas of practice, HIV is distinctive not because it is more complex than other areas of social work, but because it concentrates core challenges in a way that necessitates a socioecological approach. Several practice areas allow social workers to operate primarily within one or perhaps two socioecological levels. Child welfare work may prioritize organizational and policy/legal mandates, while mental health emphasizes intrapsychic or relational work. Engagement with PLWHA does not permit social workers to assume a narrow focus; they must concurrently address all levels of the socioecological model. The chronic nature of HIV means that many clients are involved with systems of care for years, if not decades. This long-term, resource-dependent engagement can be in sharp contrast to other areas of social work, such as child welfare or substance use, which tend to respond to acute crises and define success as case closure, reunification, or symptom reduction. HIV socializes social workers into practicing without resolution, necessitating more intense and persistent involvement with all domains of the socioecological model. Finally, the legacy of HIV, its profound impact on science, politics, and culture, disproportionate effects on marginalized communities, and continuing effects of stigma and discrimination remain relevant in contemporary social work practice. Other fields of social work have complex histories, but the findings suggest that HIV's history is unusually active, implicating PLWHA's experiences of loss, engagement with organizations, and sensitivity to policy and funding changes. The findings position HIV not merely as a context for practice, but as a developmental setting where early career social workers learn to interpret client experiences through a socioecological framework and translate knowledge into action.

Implications

Social Work Education

The findings of this study have several important implications for social work education. Participants arrived at their work with PLWHA with outdated information and received little to no education about the virus in their social work programs. As argued in this chapter, social work with PLWHA provides early career social workers a unique opportunity to develop a socioecological understanding of practice and of how oppression affects the health and wellbeing of marginalized communities. HIV is not just a medical matter, but also an area of practice that addresses every domain of the socioecological model from individual client encounters to policy advocacy. There are several wonderful resources easily accessible and available to establish core competencies for helping professionals engaged with PLWHA. The National HIV Curriculum (hiv.uw.edu) is a program of the AIDS Education and Training Center, led by the University of Washington. This comprehensive and up-to-date website offers a vast array of free resources, including primers on ART, course modules, a podcast, video mini- lectures, and symptom guides. Similarly, the HealthHIV National HIV E-Learning Training

Center (healthhiv.org/elearningcenter) also provides free programming that addresses topics of interest for anyone who wants to know more about the needs of PLWHA. Incorporating instructional materials into social work syllabi could advance the knowledge and skills of early career social workers. For historical context, documentaries such as *United in Anger: A History of ACT UP* (Hubbard, 2012) or the ACT UP Oral History Project (actuporalhistory.org), a compendium of 187 interviews with ACT UP members, would serve as valuable learning tools. Social work educators can also assign readings and case studies about HIV that touch upon contemporary issues of concern. Introducing HIV into social work classrooms would enrichen the experiences of all students, not just those interested in working with PLWHA.

The uneven and unsatisfactory experiences with supervision described by participants while in their practicum placements and post-school employment should concern social work educators. Quality supervision leads to greater job satisfaction, better client outcomes, and increased confidence in professional judgment and decision-making (Kanno & Koeske, 2010; Miehls et al., 2013; Tsui, 2004). However, Kaplan and colleagues (2025) assert that supervision remains one of the least structured and researched areas of social work practice. Concerns about the sufficiency of supervision have escalated in the post-COVID era. Many organizations remain critically understaffed, leaving senior staff with more responsibilities and less time to provide adequate supervision (Axelrad-Levy et al., 2023; Ventura et al., 2023). In this study, several participants reported that they have already assumed supervisory responsibilities. While it is not uncommon for early career social workers to find themselves in such positions, formal training in supervision is rarely included in social work curricula (Kaplan et al., 2023; Vito & Schmidt Hanbidge, 2021). Furthermore, there is a paucity of materials designed to support social workers looking to become supervisors (Hair, 2013). Students are not taught how to supervise. Given the state of the current workforce, social work schools have a responsibility to augment their courses and offer specific instruction on how to provide effective and ethical supervision.

Social work education has become increasingly focused on the proliferation and assessment of competencies (Bracy, 2018; Poulin & Matis, 2015; Regan & Detlaff, 2016). Drisko (2014) defines competencies as the knowledge, values, and skills that allow individuals to perform tasks. The Council on Social Work Education (CSWE) publishes the Educational Policy and Accreditation Standards (EPAS) (2022), which identify nine broad competencies and a set of behaviors for each competency. This framework informs the accreditation process for schools of social work at the baccalaureate, master, and doctoral level. Furthermore, the National Association of Social Workers Code of Ethics (2021) touts competence as both a core ethical principle and standard of practice. The Code states that social workers "should strive to become and remain proficient in professional practice and the performance of professional functions" (p. 25). While competencies offer shared educational expectations, measurable assessment of learning, and professional legitimacy, they imply a requirement of mastery that is fundamentally incompatible with a field where social workers find themselves practicing with incomplete information, inadequate resources, organizational uncertainty, and shifting goals (Lymbery, 2003). If early career social workers are ethically bound to be "competent", there is risk that uncertainty might be seen as shameful, rather than as an opportunity for professional growth. While competency frameworks have an important role in social work education, students also require instruction how to survive situations when they will feel uncertain, unprepared, and incompetent. Valutis (2015) argues the development of student self-awareness of discomfort in uncertain situations should be a critical learning objective. Cornish (2011) draws upon John Keats' concept of negative capability and the work of Wilfred Bion to advocate for a social work practice of "open-mindedness, receptivity, and humility" (p. 144), in contrast to a technocratic approach focused upon performance goals. Oliver (2013) introduces the language of moral distress to social work, which she describes as knowing the right thing to do but unable to act accordingly. This study reveals that practice for early career social workers engaged with PLWHA is often messy and ambiguous. Educators must support students develop necessary skills to tolerate challenging social work conditions, especially during times of political and organizational upheaval.

Social Work Practice

The implications of the findings extend beyond clinical skill acquisition. They call attention to the necessity of preparing and supporting social workers to engage with policy and organizational volatility and develop professionally within environments of high complexity and uncertainty. The following implications focus on two interrelated areas: strengthening policy and funding literacy within practice settings; and enhancing structured mentorship and professional supports for early career social workers engaged with PLWHA.

Participants described periods of fear and confusion, organizational instability affecting staffing and service continuity, and beliefs that decisions that impact their work were made without their input or the best interests of clients. These experiences suggest that policy literacy is not peripheral to social work but central to ethical practice. Several participants expressed gratitude for information about policy shifts provided by their organizations, in addition to trainings about matters such as immigration enforcement and transgender healthcare. The findings demonstrate that organizations should institutionalize structured mechanisms for translating political and policy moves into practical conversations rather than assuming social workers have the capacity to independently track these developments. This could take many forms, including regular organizational-level briefings, individual supervision sessions that specifically connect policy changes to client-level consequences, trainings on important HIV-related policy frameworks, and paid time off to participate in advocacy activities. The NASW Code of Ethics (2021) Ethical Standard 6.04 states that social workers should engage in social and political action but activism may be an additional time burden for early career social workers struggling with high caseloads and sub-standard pay.

Policy literacy has important consequences for the professional identities of early career social workers. If not adequately supported in understanding the intricacies and impact of laws and regulations, they risk misattributing structurally produced barriers as personal failures, potentially facilitating burnout and disillusionment. Not every social worker needs to become a lobbyist or policy specialist, but greater awareness of policy environments may protect against the practice challenges identified in this study.

But providing more information to early career social workers, who may already be inundated with facts and figures, is not a sufficient response in isolation. As previously noted, most participants arrived to their roles with limited knowledge of the epidemic. Their HIV education involved immersive exposure to material challenges, stigma, grief, and structural neglect. Socialization into the profession required navigation of emotionally and ethically complex situations. This labor can be difficult for new social workers. Participants shared a range of experiences with supervision, from quite positive to practically non-existent. Supervision is often focused on the details of service delivery, compliance, and performance evaluation. Early career social workers may require mentorship, broadly defined as a support network and professional connections designed to advance careers (Popowa, 2024). Mentorship can provide spaces for reflection, meaning-making, and the normalization of uncertainty that may not be possible in standard supervision. In supervision, the needs of the social worker compete with organizational and client priorities, while mentorship is often focused on a particular field of social work practice. Supervisors can leave organizations, while a mentor's availability may not be contingent on the place of employment. The Professional Association of Social Workers in HIV & AIDS (PASWHA) (pashwa.org) offers social workers at every stage of their professional development supports and community connections specifically tailored to the needs of individuals engaged with PLWHA. Organizations that serve PLWHA should consider teaming up with sibling agencies to develop formal mentorship structures that are developmentally oriented rather than evaluative. Social workers in the earliest years of the epidemic often worked across organizations to advocate, support, and uplift each other. Such collaborations could offer important spaces to nurture the next generation of social workers engaged with PLWHA. As the first generation of social workers and medical providers in this field continue to retire, there is an urgent need to capture the practice wisdom and experience that structured mentorship programs could offer (Steward et al., 2020). State and local social work organizations, such as the National Association of Social Workers (NASW), can also provide meaningful opportunities for mentorship. Together, strengthening policy literacy and cultivating mentorship offer practical pathways for sustaining early career social workers engaged with PLWHA that remain grounded in the profession's socioecological orientation.

Social Work Research

As revealed by the findings, early career social workers interpret HIV at the intersection of individual client health and wellbeing, organizational capacity, and policy unpredictability, revealing how socioecological forces shape both practice and professional formation. Yet while this study illuminates how social workers make meaning of HIV within contemporary service environments, there remain important questions about how HIV is currently understood within broader communities and how PLWHA experience an era of the epidemic marked by biomedical advancement alongside fear and uncertainty about the continued survival of programs and resources that have sustained their wellbeing. These gaps in knowledge point to critical directions for future research that extend beyond professional meaning-making to explore community narratives and lived experiences under shifting structural conditions.

Future research must examine how HIV is presently understood in diverse contexts. There exists some current research investigating contemporary attitudes and beliefs about the virus (GLAAD, 2024), but studies have not kept pace with important developments, both scientifically and socially. Community-level research, qualitative and quantitative, could explore how HIV is currently interpreted within and between generational cohorts, LGBTQ+ communities, racial and ethnic groups, and geographic areas. Other projects could examine how the chronicity framework and increasing focus on biomedical interventions align with beliefs and attitudes about the epidemic. Additionally, research might investigate existing debates concerning HIV exceptionalism and normalization, and how changing narratives impact public opinion. These lines of inquiry would ensure that research remains attuned to the lived social and political realities that influence the conceptualization of HIV.

While this study concentrates on the experiences of early career social workers, less is known about how PLWHA themselves understand and interpret contemporary organizational and policy challenges. Qualitative research with PLWHA might consider how they respond to potential changes in funding, insurance, and resource availability, while other projects could explore how organizational precarity impacts PLWHA. Research centering the voices of PLWHA is essential for understanding how broader political and social developments are experienced and negotiated in everyday life, with consequences for access to care, safety, stability, and belonging.

Social Work Policy

This study illustrates that organizational instability functions as a clinical matter. When organizations operate under threats of disruption, uncertainty and fear seep into client care. Social work policy advocacy must prioritize funding structures that support consistency, continuity of care, multi-year stability, and protection against the capricious and callous cutting of the HIV social safety net. Such work demands a comprehensive approach beyond the capacity of any one social worker or organization. Agencies that serve the needs of PLWHA must collaborate to ensure that the voices of clients and frontline workers inform decision-making at all levels of government. Outside advocacy groups, including ACT UP, would be natural partners in such campaigns. These efforts would represent an ethical responsibility vital to both the continued wellbeing of PLWHA and the long-term sustainability of the social work workforce engaged with these clients.

Activism should not focus exclusively upon the biomedical aspects of the epidemic. Participants consistently described that viral suppression was difficult and insufficient in the absence of housing, transportation access, regular income, and mental health and substance use services. If success in social work with PLWHA is measured solely through biomedical markers such as decreased viral loads and higher CD4 counts, structural vulnerabilities risk being minimized. As the experiences of participants make clear, medical progress is highly dependent on the multitude of health, material, and social resources that support medication adherence. HIV policy must continue to support and incorporate housing stabilization programs, adequate financial support for transportation systems, and robust and readily accessible mental health and substance use care. When debates concerning the end of the epidemic are isolated from the structural contexts where the virus resides, important policy objectives will be undermined, thus prolonging and perhaps deteriorating the current state of affairs.

Limitations and Strengths

There are several limitations to this study. Important epistemological and methodological issues have been raised about qualitative research methods. The emphasis on smaller, purposive samples provides depth, yet findings may be represented in ways that raise concerns about generalizability and representativeness (Johnson et al., 2020; Young & Casey, 2019). Since qualitative analysis relies heavily on researcher interpretation, findings are vulnerable to selective attention and confirmation bias (Mackieson et al., 2019; Noble & Smith, 2025). Inconsistent standards have led to wide variation in how rigor is reported in studies, making it challenging to evaluate study quality or compare findings across projects (Levitt et al., 2018). Qualitative approaches may also suffer from social desirability bias, or a mismatch between a participant's experience and how they present that reality to the researcher (Bergen & Labonté, 2020). Interpretative Phenomenological Analysis (IPA), the chosen method of data analysis for this study, has been subjected to critique for limitations in rigor, potential for bias, and lack of epistemological clarity (Brocki & Wearden, 2006; Noon, 2018; Pringle et al., 2011; Tuffour, 2017). These concerns highlight the importance of approaching qualitative inquiry, and IPA specifically, with sustained reflexivity and methodological transparency.

As discussed in Chapter 3, this study incorporated multiple safeguards to enhance credibility, transparency, and integrity within the selected qualitative research methods. Throughout all stages of data collection and analysis, I drafted extensive memoranda detailing participant observations, my reactions to the data, connections to the conceptual framework guiding the study, and ideas for future directions. This reflexive approach kept me grounded in the data while acknowledging the emotional impact of the research process. The iterative coding process demanded by IPA required close, sustained engagement with each transcript, tracking how participants made sense of their experiences while testing my emerging interpretations. Regular conversations with social work colleagues offered fresh perspectives and suggestions that sharpened my analysis. These strategies acknowledged the subjectivity of the work and made the methodology more accountable.

Sampling and recruitment proved to be one of the biggest challenges of this project and an important limitation. The inclusion criteria for "early career social worker" was intentionally broadened to include individuals with up to ten years of post-MSW experience in hopes of spurring engagement. While there is no agreed definition as to "early career", studies have operationalized this concept to include social workers with experience of one year or less (Bates et al., 2010), two years or less (Lim et al., 2025; Neill et al., 2025), or five years or less (McCulloch et al., 2024; Petersén, 2024). No studies have been located which take such an expansive definition of "early career" as adopted in this project. Six of the twenty-two participants (27.3%) reported having more than 5 years post-MSW experience, some of whom were on the cusp of exclusion from the study. The inclusion criteria reflect the lack of consensus in the book and acknowledge that professional development may extend beyond the first years of employment. A review of the transcripts demonstrated no significant differences in the themes raised by participants with less than five years and participants with more than five years of experience. Furthermore, the specialized nature of this area of social work practice necessitated a wider inclusion criteria.

Recruitment difficulties may have contributed to a more heterogeneous sample than advisable. More diverse qualitative samples risk generating findings that are diffuse or underdeveloped (Levitt et al., 2018; Malterud et al., 2016). Within this sample, there are notable differences in geographic residence, areas of practice, and years of post-MSW experience. Rather than ignore this variation, I explain and analyze where appropriate. For instance, I note how social workers focused on mental health concerns often had very different encounters with their PLWHA clients compared to participants engaged in medical case management. The demonstrated similarities among participants' experiences ultimately sustains the coherence of the study's findings and interpretations.

Finally, this study is affected by temporal and contextual limitations. The experiences of early career social workers engaged with PLWHA may be vastly different from those of veteran practitioners, especially those employed during the worst years of the epidemic. Data collection took place at a time (December 2024-April 2025) of considerable political changes, anchoring this study's findings to the historical moment. As policy and organizational volatility may increase or subside, and with continuing biomedical advancements in the treatment of HIV, the work of this study might be time-bound. The findings should be considered as an interpretive account situated in a particular professional generation and political moment.

Despite these limitations, this study offers an in-depth, original, and theoretically framed exploration of how early career social workers engaged with PLWHA make meaning of their work during times of uncertainty and instability. By bridging participants' meaning-making processes with structural forces and integrating socioecological and life course theories with lived professional experiences, this research moves beyond siloed analysis to offer a multi-layered account of social work with PLWHA. The five chapters of findings, each rooted in a domain of the socioecological model, are replete with extensive quotations by participants, centering their voices. Additionally, the research is timely and relevant, providing insights that can guide curriculum development, organizational policy, and advocacy efforts. This study makes a clear and meaningful contribution to social work book.

Chapter 10
Conclusion

This book explores the lived experiences of early career social workers engaged with PLWHA and employs the socioecological model as the conceptual framework to describe how they make sense and meaning of their efforts on behalf of clients and organizations. The research question centering this work is: "What are the experiences of early career social workers engaged with PLWHA?" Twenty-two individuals participated in a qualitative research study that employed semi-structured interviews. Data were analyzed using interpretative phenomenological analysis (IPA).

In Chapter 2, I provide an overview of the history of HIV in the United States, the current state of the epidemic, and social work's vital role in addressing one of the most consequential health, social, scientific, and political challenges of the modern era. This background is necessary to situate the present study within broader historical, structural, and professional contexts and present the rich, complicated legacy inherited by today's social workers. I offer a modified socioecological model as the conceptual framework guiding the study and depict its historical origins and application to the experiences of social workers and other helping professionals. The socioecological model is a strong choice because of its alignment with social work values and disciplinary identity and its utility in connecting individual-level experiences to structural forces, and vice versa. Life course theory supplements the socioecological model by introducing a temporal dimension that attends to how personal and professional experiences unfold across the life course.

In Chapter 3, I detail the methodological decisions and dilemmas encountered during the research process and describe sampling and recruitment, data collection, data analysis, and considerations of rigor, trustworthiness, and ethical issues. A reflexivity statement provides important context as to how my identities, experiences, and perspectives shape my approach to the work. Chapters 4 through 8 present the findings of the study, with each chapter concentrated upon a domain of the socioecological model. Chapter 4 focuses on individual-level factors impacting early career social workers in their engagement with PLWHA, including their journeys to the social work profession, previous knowledge about the virus, experiences in social work school and practicum placements, knowledge and skills gained, self-care strategies, and the personal impact of the work. Chapter 5 examines the interpersonal factors of the socioecological model, looking at how social workers' conceptualize their clients' HIV care, challenges and barriers, the role of relationship, generational differences, the salience of HIV, and matters related to self-disclosure.

Chapter 6 shifts to organizational contexts experienced by early career social workers engaged with PLWHA. Relevant findings include participants' interest in their organizations, job responsibilities and satisfaction, supervisory experiences and intra-organizational collaboration, the role of the organization in the lives of clients, perceived benefits of an HIV diagnosis, and organizational responses to current event. Chapter 7 looks at community-level factors such as inter-organizational collaborations and the phenomenon of stigma and its relevance to social work practice with PLWHA. Chapter 8 concludes the findings chapters by examining the policy and social factors of the socioecological model, consisting of client and social worker concerns about current events, HIV as a matter of social concern, the continued need for HIV-specific programs, understanding of systems, HIV exceptionalism, and the future of social work with

PLWHA.

Chapter 9 presents three overarching themes that unify the study's findings. The first theme considers how early career social workers, many of whom have no memory of the worst years of the epidemic, make sense of HIV in their work with PLWHA. The second theme focuses on the practice of social work during times of uncertainty and instability. The third theme presents HIV as a social work lens and site for professional development and socialization. Each theme is closely related to the findings at each domain of the socioecological model. Implications of the findings are discussed in relation to social work education, practice, research and policy. The chapter ends with a reflection on the limitations and strengths of the study.

www.ingramcontent.com/pod-product-compliance
Lightning Source LLC
LaVergne TN
LVHW050805061126
851857LV00012B/683